Prescription Drug Abuse

Mark J. Estren, Ph.D.

RONIN

Berkeley, CA

Prescription Drug Abuse

Mark J. Estren, Ph.D.

Prescription Drug Abuse
Copyright 2013: Mark J. Estren
ISBN: 978-1-57951-168-5

Published by
Ronin Publishing, Inc.
PO Box 22900
Oakland, CA 94609
www.roninpub.com

Production:
  Cover: Brian Groppe
  Book design: Beverly A. Potter
  Editor: Beverly A. Potter

Credits:
  Page 13: Photo by Darren Lewis.
  Page 37: Courtesy National Cancer Institute.
  Page 63: Photo by Bill Branson, courtesy National
    Cancer Institute.
  Page 75: Photo by Vera Kratochvil.
  Page 99: Photo by Linda Bartlett, courtesy National
    Cancer Institute.
  Page 121: Courtesy National Library of Medicine.

Library of Congress Card Number: 2013940511

Distributed to the book trade by PGW/Perseus

In Memory of Dr. G. S. Goldman

My emphasis on the importance of putting patients' needs first even in the face of an admitted societal problem reflects the influence of my father-in-law, psychoanalyst George S. Goldman, M.D. (1906-2008). He and I share a Columbia University connection: I earned my master's in journalism from Columbia, while George was the longtime Director of the Columbia University Psychoanalytic Clinic for Training & Research.

As co-editor in 1965 of *Developments in Psychoanalysis at Columbia University*, George wrote with mild disapproval of "the reluctance of many analysts to accept change," looking ahead to a "new generation which will shape and mold the future," young psychoanalysts who would "maintain their flair for the experimental and exploratory" and who "have learned the necessity and appreciation of tolerance—tolerance of differences with which they disagree, and tolerance amongst their critics."

In the 21st century, where tolerance so often seems quaint, George's hopeful views are worth remembering, applicable as they are not just to psychiatry, not just to medicine, but to human relationships in general. George understood the importance of listening—someone who practiced psychoanalysis until age 85 would have to!—and of flexibility, but also the importance of knowing when *not* to be flexible. He never compromised his focus on patients or his belief that the efficacy of talk therapy was far greater than that of behavior-modifying medications. He was not happy to see psychoanalysis moving toward a medication-focused model—and would not be surprised at the "collateral damage" that prescription drugs have inflicted on society.

Other Books by Dr. Mark J. Estren

A History of Underground Comics

Statins: Miraculous or Misguided?

Healing Hormones

Table of Contents

1: The Depth of the Pain............................9

2: Creating Homelessness............................18

3: Attack on Pseudoephedrine............................32

4: Government on Opioids............................40

5: Government Responds............................47

6: Disposal & Enforcement............................57

7: Victimizing the Victims............................65

8: Washington State's Rx............................71

9: Abuse Beyond Opioids............................79

10: Abuse Sneaks In............................87

11: How Abuse Happens............................99

12: Helping without Guilt............................108

13: Love and Intervention............................117

Bibliography & References............................129

Author Bio............................137

1

The Depth of the Pain

While most major causes of preventable death are declining in the United States, drugs are an exception. The death toll from drugs has doubled in the last decade: they now claim a life every fourteen minutes. Drugs kill more people than traffic accidents.

Fueling the surge in deaths are prescription pain and anxiety drugs that are potent, highly addictive and especially dangerous when combined with one another or with other drugs or alcohol. Among the most commonly abused are OxyContin®, Vicodin®, Xanax®, Soma® and Fentanyl®—a painkiller that comes in the form of patches and lollipops and is a hundred times more powerful than morphine. These drugs now cause more deaths than heroin and cocaine combined. And they are almost certainly in your medicine cabinet.

At some point, everyone needs pain medicine—from aspirin or Tylenol® to prescription-strength opioids. At some point, everyone suffers from anxiety—in many cases, seriously enough to need prescription-strength medicines. But the people using the medicines, and sometimes the doctors prescribing them, do not know all the drugs' dangers. And in this case, what you don't know can hurt you—even kill you.

Predictably, the government has stepped in. The result is that patients have been caught between the proverbial "rock and a hard place." More than one-

third of Americans have chronic pain and need medicines
that can potentially be abused. Because of government
regulations and restrictions, they
What you don't may not be able to get those drugs;
know can hurt if they do get them, they are at risk
you—even kill you. of becoming addicted. More than
one-fifth of Americans take at least
one drug for a psychological disorder—and here, too, the
desperately needed medicines may not be available, and
can be dangerous when patients are able to obtain them.

The stories of prescription-drug fatalities are heart-
rending. Overdose victims range in age and circum-
stance from teenagers who pop pills to get a heroin-like
high to middle-aged working men and women who take
medications prescribed for strained backs and bad knees
and become addicted. A 19-year-old Army recruit,
who had just passed his military physical, died after he
took a handful of Xanax® and painkillers while party-
ing with friends. A groom, anxious over his upcoming
wedding, overdosed on a cocktail of prescription drugs.
A teenage honors student overdosed on painkillers
that her father had left in his medicine cabinet from a
surgery years earlier. A toddler was orphaned after both
parents overdosed on prescription drugs a few months
apart. A grandmother suffering from chronic back pain
apparently forgot she'd already taken her daily regimen
of pills and ended up double dosing—and dying.

The Greater Danger

IN SOME WAYS, prescription drugs are more dangerous
than illicit ones, because users don't have their guard
up. People feel they are safer with prescription drugs because they come from pharmacies and are prescribed by
doctors. Younger people believe they are safer because

they see their parents taking them. These medicines don't have the same stigma as street narcotics.

These drugs do enormous good, which rarely gets as much attention as the relatively small amount of harm they do—which, of course, is not to say that the harm is small to families affected. Because news reports focus on the exceptions—the addicts, the abusers, the people who die from legal medications—the media miss a much larger and societally more significant situation. Just outside the headlines and off the front pages are stories that tug even harder at the heartstrings than ones about overdoses and unwarranted deaths: people in terrible pain who cannot get legal relief because the government won't allow them to have it; doctors trying to help desperate patients and, as a result, finding themselves branded as drug dealers; pharmacists refusing legitimate prescriptions out of fear that the government will target them for pushing pills.

How It Started

THE SEEDS of the prescription-drug-abuse problem were planted well over a decade ago by well-meaning efforts by doctors to mitigate suffering, as well as aggressive sales campaigns by pharmaceutical manufacturers. The problem the drugs address is real and growing. Serious, chronic pain affects at least one hundred-sixteen million Americans each year, many of whom are inadequately treated by the health-care system, according to the Institute of Medicine. The reasons for long-lasting pain are many, from cancer and multiple sclerosis to back pain and arthritis, and the chronic suffering costs the United States five hundred-sixty billion to six hundred thirty-five billion dollars each year in medical bills, lost productivity and missed work.

Yet pain patients have long been viewed with skepticism and suspicion, rather than understanding—presenting a barrier to care. Rising rates of prescription drug misuse, addiction and overdose have led to the establishment of legal and regulatory barriers, such as prescription databases, that can prevent legitimate pain patients from getting much-needed drugs. The result is a culture of abuse on both sides: abuse when individuals who do not genuinely need these medicines seek them, and abuse of patients that occurs when people who do need pain medications cannot get them because physicians won't prescribe them or the state and federal governments have regulatory barriers.

Making matters worse is the disturbing fact that the media and political establishments devote considerable attention to painkiller abuse and addiction—but very little to chronic pain, which affects a far greater number of people. About nine point three percent of the population has drug or alcohol problems serious enough to require treatment, while severe chronic pain affects more than three times as many people—at least one in three Americans. Yet two national institutes are devoted to the research of addiction—the National Institute on Alcoholism and Alcohol Abuse and the National Institute on Drug Abuse—while there is no National Institute on Pain at all.

The media and political establishments pay little attention to chronic pain.

The Sufferers

IN RECENT YEARS, health-care professionals have increasingly been saying that patients in hospices and nursing homes are suffering needlessly because they cannot get pain medicines. The reason is a combination of regulatory changes, periodic manufacturing snags and physicians' reluctance to prescribe the drugs in light of a growing number of abuses of opioid painkillers, such as oxycodone and hydrocodone.

For example, Shane Craycraft, administrator at a nursing home in Middleton, Ohio, at one point noted that residents were waiting two or three days before receiving pain-relief medication, a delay that he said was "significantly affecting pain management." A hospice nurse in Greensboro, North Carolina, Leslie Millikin, also saw an access problem when the supply of liquid morphine, a crucial pain medicine, was extremely limited. "If [patients] can't swallow, they need this," said Millikin. Why couldn't they get it? First, the Food and Drug Administration entered an order against a key drug manufacturer, limiting the supply of morphine. Then the FDA told several manufacturers to stop making several pain-relief drugs because the medications had been developed so long ago that they had not gone through the agency's approval process—and one of the targeted drugs was a form of liquid morphine.

In that particular case, patient advocates persuaded the agency to keep that specific medicine on the market, citing a hardship on terminally ill patients. But the FDA has never acknowledged anything wrong with its basic approach—which, if applied to other medicines, could lead to taking aspirin off the market, since it also

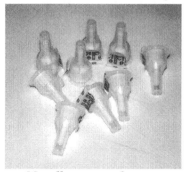

Needles in packaging

was developed too long ago, in 1897, to have gone
through FDA approval requirements: the FDA was not
established in its present form until 1930.

Attempted Balance

THERE IS AN APPARENT REASONABLENESS of efforts to
balance the legitimate needs of pain patients with law-
enforcement determination to root out abuse of prescription painkillers. And no one sounds more reasonable than the medical professionals who work for the
federal government. Wilson M. Compton, MD, director
of the Division of Epidemiology, Services and Prevention Research at the National Institute on Drug Abuse,
first called it "a national priority" to prevent abuse of
prescription painkillers, then added, "Our goal would
be to minimize the abuse and addiction while making
sure they [opioids] remain available to combat pain and
suffering."

It sounds good, but it does not work that way. In
practice, as the privately run American Pain Foundation, a consumer advocacy group, has pointed out, legitimate patients are having far greater trouble than in
the past in obtaining pain
The lack of government   drugs. And Judy Lentz,
empathy for pain   CEO of the Hospice and
patients is striking.   Palliative Nurses Association, said that a survey of
ninteen hundred hospice nurses discovered that more
than half "identified tremendous problems" in access to
pain medications, even for "people in the last hours of
life." Lentz said, "We don't disagree with what [govern-
ment officials] are trying to do, [but] we want them to

understand the consequences to our vulnerable population."

But they don't understand. That is not their job.
The lack of government empathy for pain patients
is striking. Gary Boggs, a special agent for the Drug
Enforcement Agency, known as the DEA, said, "We
certainly don't want the patients to go without pain
medication." But he quickly focused on the government's real orientation: restricting supply by making
sure correct procedures are followed at all times. Nurses
in nursing homes often improperly phone in painkiller
prescriptions using information on a patient chart,
said Boggs, and while this practice is fine for hospitals,
which are DEA-registered, it is improper for unregis-
tered nursing homes to do similar nurse-ordering.

But patients discharged from hospitals often arrive
at nursing homes without medication—frequently on
Friday nights, when it is hard to track down a doctor to
authorize a prescription, said Sandra Fitzler, senior director of clinical services for the American Health Care
Association. And physicians often do not visit nursing
homes on a daily basis. "This has created a mess," Fitzler
said.

That is an understatement. The government itself—which, after all, is not monolithic but is an as-
semblage of multiple parts, not all of which know what
other parts are doing or
are in agreement about *This has created a mess.*
policies and proce-   —Sandra Fitzler
dures—is at cross-pur-   American Health Care Assoc.
poses when it comes to
pain medicines. At one point, two Democratic senators,
Herb Kohl of Wisconsin and Sheldon Whitehouse of
Rhode Island, both members of the U.S. Senate Special

Committee on Aging, sent a letter to Attorney General Eric Holder urging prompt access to prescription pain medication. "Significant numbers of long-term-care and hospice patients may not be receiving much-needed pain relief and other medications...in a timely manner," the senators wrote, linking delays in delivering the medicines to stepped-up DEA enforcement of long-term-care and hospice medication practices. But nothing came of the letter, because pain patients are an amorphous, ever-changing group with no effective central voice in the government—while "everybody" agrees that the DEA must root out prescription drug abuse by stopping the doctors who make most of it possible.

"Everybody," though, is wrong. Only one-fifth of people who misuse opioid painkillers get their drugs exclusively from doctors—and sixty-nine percent of abusers never obtain *any* drugs from *any* medical sources. William Clark Becker, MD, of Yale University, looked at data from the annual National Household Survey on Drug Use and Health between 2006 and 2008, collecting information on more than three thousand people over age eighteen who reported having

Pain patients are an amorphous, ever-changing group with no effective central voice in the government.

taken an opioid painkiller that either was not prescribed for them or that they used for nonmedical reasons in the last month. The study, published in *Archives of Internal Medicine*, found overwhelmingly that most opioid misusers were not being treated for pain and had obtained their drugs from friends, family or dealers, not doctors.

Opioids and Cocaine

BUT SURELY DOCTORS ARE RESPONSIBLE for patients developing drug problems in the first place and must therefore be far more carefully watched and regulated? Again, no. Research has been done on this, too, and it turns out that fewer than three percent of people become addicted this way. In fact, eighty percent of OxyContin® misusers have previously taken cocaine, which certainly suggests that their addiction is unlikely to have originated from being legitimately prescribed an opioid for pain.

Despite the research, though, government efforts to fight opioid misuse are focused almost exclusively on trying to get doctors to write fewer prescriptions and using databases to track patients' medical records and doctors' prescribing habits.

A genuinely balanced approach—and one more likely to be successful—would be to focus, first, on what drives people with drug problems to seek out opioids; and, second, on supply sources other than doctors, including foreign drug companies, dealers, and theft from factories, friends and family.

This would deal both with the problem of pain-killer misuse and with that of legitimate pain patients not being able to get drugs. It would be a balanced and nuanced approach—but the government is not noted for balance or nuance. So instead we have a policy that intimidates health-care professionals and leaves some of the most highly vulnerable patients of all in unremitting physical agony. And it is by no means the first policy with such serious unintended consequences.

2

Creating Homelessness

Government attempts to prevent the abuse of pain-killers and anti-psychotic medications have unintended consequences—and this is scarcely the first time that well-intended government policies, which look good when written, have caused severe hardship for individuals and for society at large. With the stated intention of treating the mentally ill more humanely, the government implemented a policy called *deinstitutionalization*—the removal of patients from mental hospitals and their integration into the community—and ended up creating a permanent underclass of homeless people.

Deinstitutionalization was well-meaning on its face in its attempt to be responsive to genuine concerns about the horrible treatment often accorded the mentally ill in the past. The policy relied heavily on the use of medications as an alternative to forced confinement. But, far from helping mentally ill people to be integrated back into society, deinstitutionalization *caused* the massive problem of homelessness—which the government has subsequently spent decades, and huge amounts of taxpayer money, *trying to solve*.

Proponents of deinstitutionalization traced the problem of treating the mentally ill to the 19th century, a time when mental illness was considered a moral failing or the result of demonic possession—think of all those Victorian novels featuring crazed relatives hidden away in attics. In 1868, Elizabeth Packard founded the Anti-Insane Asylum Society after she was released from an asylum to which her husband had committed her: men who were unable to get a divorce could have their wives committed to get them out of the way. But Packard's pamphlets, although filled with shocking details, produced no public reaction in light of then-current beliefs about mental illness.

In 1887, investigative journalist Nellie Bly got herself admitted to an asylum and reported on the terrible conditions there in a book called *Ten Days in a Mad-House*. Even today, passages from Bly's book resonate with Dickensian horror:

Soon after my advent a girl called Urena Little-Page was brought in. She was, as she had been born, silly, and her tender spot was, as with many sensible women, her age. She claimed eighteen, and would grow very angry if told to the contrary. The nurses were not long in finding this out, and then they teased her.

"Urena," said Miss Grady, "the doctors say that you are thirty-three instead of eighteen," and the other nurses laughed. They kept up this until the simple creature began to yell and cry, saying she wanted to go home and that everybody treated her badly. After they had gotten all the amusement out of her they wanted and she was crying, they began to scold and tell her to keep quiet. She grew more hysterical every moment until they pounced upon her and slapped her face and knocked her head in a lively fashion. This made the poor creature cry the more, and so they choked her. Yes, actually choked her. Then they dragged her out to the closet, and I heard her terri-

*fied cries hush into smothered ones. After several
hours' absence she returned to the sitting-room, and
I plainly saw the marks of their fingers on her throat
for the entire day.*

*This punishment seemed to awaken their desire to
administer more. They returned to the sitting-room
and caught hold of an old gray-haired woman whom
I have heard addressed both as Mrs. Grady and Mrs.
O'Keefe. She was insane, and she talked almost
continually to herself and to those near her. She
never spoke very loud, and at the time I speak of was
sitting harmlessly chattering to herself. They grabbed
her, and my heart ached as she cried:*

"For God sake, ladies, don't let them beat me."

*"Shut up, you hussy!" said Miss Grady as she
caught the woman by her gray hair and dragged her
shrieking and pleading from the room. She was also
taken to the closet, and her cries grew lower and
lower, and then ceased.*

Not Yet

THE TIME WAS NOT RIGHT for effective muckrak-
ing about mental health. Later books, such as *A Mind
That Found Itself*, written in 1908 by Clifford W. Beers,
garnered somewhat more attention, but it was not really until the 1948 movie, *The Snake Pit* with Olivia de
Havilland, that the public in the United States took
notice of the horrors of life in the places known as
insane asylums.

Even with the conditions revealed, it took a conflu-
ence of events in the 1950s and 1960s to bring about
deinstitutionalization. Overcrowding of asylums, budget

cuts during times of economic trouble and war, ongoing reports of abuse and death of patients, and the rise of disability activism were some elements.

Then Came Drugs

IT WAS THE CREATION in 1950 of chlorpromazine, sold as Thorazine®, Largactil® or Megaphen®, and the subsequent development of other antipsychotics, that set the stage for deinstitutionalization. The use of chlorpromazine quickly led to decreases in electroconvulsive therapy, often called "shock treatment," and in psychosurgery, such as lobotomy—the surgery that Nurse Ratched ordered done to Murphy in *One Flew Over the Cuckoo's Nest*.

Chlorpromazine provided, or seemed to provide, a less-expensive, more patient-friendly solution to mental illness—and a way to integrate the mentally ill into society at large. Arguments for deinstitutionalization flourished in the 1950s and gained significant additional impetus in the early 1960s, partly because President Kennedy revealed the mental illness in his own family—his oldest sister, Rosemary Kennedy, had been lobotomized—and partly because the anti-authoritarian mindset of the decade made centralized institutions such as asylums seem not only anachronistic but also inherently dehumanizing.

The stated goal of deinstitutionalization was integration of the mentally ill into society as productive members. To succeed, it required a devolution of care to community centers, including such factors as supported and supervised housing and team intervention. It was assumed that, in these settings, the mentally ill would go on taking their chlorpromazine or other drugs. Issues such as noncompliance with drug regimens, lack of coordination of local services, the complex individual needs of the mentally ill, and the difficulty of integrating patients with their own families—because of the families' resistance or the patients' own refusal—were never considered or were downplayed.

Lack of Support

THE RESULT WAS that people were released from asylums without sufficient preparation or support. The government strongly advocated the use of medications to stabilize, if not cure, mental illness. Insurance carriers went along enthusiastically with deinstitutionalization, since the costs of ongoing psychiatric care and hospitalization were far higher than

It was the development of antipsychotic drugs that made deinstitutionalization possible.

those of prescribing medicine. The result was the rapid, permanent loss of thousands of hospital beds—and the insidious creation of a new, permanent underclass euphemistically called "the homeless."

There is nothing new about homelessness in the United States. But deinstitutionalization changed its character. Before mental hospitals emptied their patients into the streets, homelessness was generally a temporary phenomenon, as when the Great Depression led to creation of a subculture of "hobos" wandering the country looking for nonexistent jobs. Generally, though, as the economy improved, these people found jobs—and homes. True, there were areas of major cities where hobos—or "bums"—lived year-round: the Bowery in New York and Tenderloin in San Francisco, for example. But these were isolated pockets of cities; since deinstitutionalization, the homeless are much more widespread.

Wishful Lawmaking

WHAT WENT WRONG? During the Kennedy presidency, with increasing pressure from reformers and the backing of a sympathetic president, Congress passed the Community Mental Health Centers Act in 1963. The law sought to create a system of mental health centers that would focus on preventive, community-based outpatient care as an alternative to institutionalization of the mentally ill in state mental hospitals. States liked this plan for community care—and the promise of funds to support it, which offered states relief from the huge financial costs of housing the mentally ill in hospitals.

Lillian B. Rubin neatly encapsulated officials' reactions in an article in *Dissent* magazine: "State and local officials spoke

D einstitutionalization was undertaken without sufficient preparation or support.

the language of mental health advocacy and community care, but they acted on their concern for fiscal policy."

So without waiting for the promised funding of care centers for the newly deinstitutionalized, governments became strong advocates of the concept. They transferred tens of thousands of mentally ill women and men into communities that had no way to support their care. Compounding the problem was the fact that many of these people had spent years in confinement and as a result had few independent-living skills. The money to implement the well-intentioned deinstitutionalization plan never appeared.

The Vietnam War, tax revolts and shifting governmental priorities got in the way. The result was devastating, not only for the mentally ill but also for the professionals who cared for them—or tried to. Rubin quotes
one such professional as saying, "We had no choice but
to turn people out into the street. ...The state hospital,
the place of last resort, was gone; there were no halfway
homes, no treatment programs, nothing."

But deinstitutionalization continued, an unstoppa-
ble steamroller that led in relatively short order to the
closure of nearly half the hospitals in the United States
and a dramatic reduction of bed capacity in the ones
that remained. The effect on patients? Tens of thousands—no one really knows how many—were
sent out into the streets, unsupported and unable to
care for themselves in a society that had turned its back
on them.

The money to implement the well-intentioned deinstitutionalization plan never appeared.

Just Give Meds

IN THE ABSENCE OF mental hospitals as places of last
resort, the government established drugs as the primary
method of treating the mentally ill. But the medicines
themselves had unintended consequences. A whole
new set of issues emerged because of side effects ranging from weight gain and blurred vision to physically
debilitating motor difficulties. Thus, thousands of deinstitutionalized patients were thrown right back into the
health-care system—or onto the streets as a permanent
class of homeless.

Nowadays, according to Rubin, the best treatment that any mentally ill homeless person is likely to get "is a bed to rest in just long enough for the doctors to find the right drug regimen to stabilize a crisis." And then what? It is back to the homeless camp, because the community offers no services, no follow-up, and no place to live.

In 2007, when Rubin's article appeared, the estimate was that even though a number of people who would once have been institutionalized had been taken in by their families or absorbed into group homes and charity living spaces, some five hudred thousand of the seven hundred fifty thousand homeless Americans were living in shelters or on the streets. They were locked in the institutions of their own *The treatment of last resort—and* mental illnesses *also, often, of first resort—was* even though *medication.* the bricks-and-mortar institutions designed to help them—and admittedly to confine them—no longer existed. Although this "virtual epidemic" has many complex causes, Rubin and others attribute it, in large part, to two milestones of public policy: the Housing Act of 1949, which initiated urban renewal, and the Community Mental Health Centers Act of 1963, which attempted to reform the mental health system.

If there were seven hundred fifty thousand or so homeless in the first decade of the century, the number, according to most observers, has continued to grow. In the words of Paul Appelbaum, MD, a professor of psychiatry, medicine and law at the Columbia University College of Physicians and Surgeons in New York, "The state of the mental health system in this country is really pitiful. Most people would not even dignify it with the term 'system.'"

The collapse of the well-intentioned notion of deinstitutionalization in favor of a medication-based regimen of mental-illness treatment was described in *Madness in the Streets: How Psychiatry and the Law Abandoned the Mentally Ill*. According to authors Rael Jean Isaac and Virginia C. Armat, a combination of potent cultural and political changes in the 1960s caused deinstitutionalization and then prevented those with the power to deal with the mentally ill from "confronting and ending this disgrace to our society."

The 1960s were a turbulent time for all forms of authority, which was often considered synonymous with oppression. Anti-authoritarianism was a factor behind a concerted attack on the psychiatric establishment. Activists asserted that mental illness was a myth—those labeled mentally ill were merely "different" and were unfairly stigmatized as a result. Rallying behind seminal anti-psychiatric works such as Thomas Szasz' *The Myth of Mental Illness*, activists argued that those with real mental "problems" could effectively be treated in the community—because integrating people who thought and behaved "differently" into the mainstream would be far better than isolating them and treating them like freaks, as if there were something "wrong" with them.

According to Isaac and Armat, psychiatry "buckled under the attack, accepting these misguided and untested notions, and now our society offers no real response to people in need of help."

The 1960s brought huge enthusiasm for a kind of civil-rights approach to social problems in general. In the case of mental illness, what that meant was that it became nearly impossible to give someone medical help without his or her consent—no matter how desperate families and others might be to try to protect the person and those with whom he or she might come in contact. "A short walk through any American community today reveals the utter failure of these policies," write Isaac and Armat. "Our sidewalks and parks have become open-air mental wards—but without treatment for their inmates."

Of course, treatment in the form of medicine *is* available, but the mentally ill cannot be forced to accept meds—or to take them if they do accept them. The standard for temporarily hospitalizing and forcibly medicating someone is that he or she must be a clear and present danger to himself or herself—or to others. That is virtually impossible to prove until the person tries to commit suicide or physically attacks someone

> *Now our society offers no real response to people in need of help.*
>
> —Rael Jean Isaac and Virginia C. Armat
> *Madness in the Streets*

else. Once again, there is an unintended consequence here: treating the mentally ill as simply "different" gives them the right to refuse medication that could help them. And preventing them from being shut away in institutions takes away the right of many city residents to walk down the street unworried and unmolested.

Branded for Life

DESPITE ALL OF THIS, it is important not to paint the proponents of deinstitutionalization with too broad a brush or act as if there was some conspiracy afoot to destroy a mental-health system that was working pretty well, despite occasional excesses. The system was *not* working well. A series of famous, if controversial, experiments by psychologist David Rosenhan in 1973 showed how eight perfectly normal people could be branded for life as mental patients. In the study, they claimed a brief instance of auditory hallucinations— which led to their admission to mental hospitals for an average of nineteen days. To be discharged, they had to "admit" to having a mental illness and agree to take antipsychotic drugs after being released.

The unintended consequences of government policies are just that—unintended. But they are also extremely far-reaching, and have had major effects on the entire society. In 1955, there were 558,239 severely mentally ill patients in public psychiatric hospitals in the United States, which then had a total population of 164 million. By 1994, this number had been reduced to only 71,619—a drop of 486,620 patients—while the nation's population had grown to 260 million. If statistical trends had held up—that is, if there had been the same proportion of patients per population in public mental hospitals in 1994 as there had been in 1955—then the patient total would have been 885,010 in 1994. So to get a fair picture of the significance of deinstitutionalization, we must look at the difference between the expected number of patients, 885,010, and the actual number, 71,619. That means that 813,391 patients—or ninty-two percent of the people—who would have been living in public psychiatric hospitals in 1955 were not living there in 1994. The loss of patient population—and of beds for treating the mentally ill—is now irreversible.

The mental health system that existed before deinstitutionalization was not working well.

The Homeless Today

WHO ARE THE HOMELESS NOW? E. Fuller Torrey, MD, explains in *Out of the Shadows: Confronting America's Mental Illness Crisis* that most of those released during deinstitutionalization were severely mentally ill—between fifty and sixty percent diagnosed with schizophrenia, another ten to fifteen percent with manic-depressive illness and severe depression, and an additional ten to fifteen percent with organic brain diseases, including epilepsy, strokes, Alzheimer's disease, and brain damage secondary to trauma.

Other patients who had been in public psychiatric hospitals had such conditions as mental retardation with psychosis, autism and other psychiatric disorders of childhood, and alcoholism and drug addiction—with brain damage.

The result, Torrey says, is that "deinstitutionalization has helped create the mental illness crisis." How? By releasing people from public psychiatric hospitals without consistently following up by giving them the medicine and rehabilitation services they need to live successfully in the community. And then deinstitutionalization made things even worse, because

> *Deinstitutionalization has helped create the mental illness crisis.*

now that the public psychiatric beds are gone, they are not available for people who have become mentally ill since deinstitutionalization. Torrey estimates that approximately 2.2 million severely mentally ill people do not receive *any* psychiatric treatment.

The underlying concept of deinstitutionalization was that severe mental illness should be treated in the least restrictive setting. President Jimmy Carter's Commission on Mental Health, in 1978, explained the foundation of this ideology—and it was ideology, not science or medicine—as having "the objective of maintaining the greatest degree of freedom, self-determination, autonomy, dignity, and integrity of body, mind, and spirit for the individual while he or she participates in treatment or receives services."

Even if the Carter Commission's goal has been realized—at least partially—Torrey concludes that "for a substantial minority, however, deinstitutionalization has been a psychiatric Titanic." Instead of what the government called lives of "dignity, and integrity of body, mind, and spirit," these people receive only enough self-determination to choose among soup kitchens. The least-restrictive setting for them is all too often, according to Torrey, "a cardboard box, a jail cell, or a terror-filled existence plagued by both real and imaginary enemies."

> *For a substantial minority... deinstitutionalization has been a psychiatric Titanic.*
> —E. Fuller Torrey, M.D.

Real-World Results

NO MATTER HOW GOOD THE RATIONALE of government programs, they inevitably have unintended consequences—including the creation of a nationwide "homeless problem" as well as a treatment regimen that relies on antipsychotic medications that have become far more effective over the years but that still have numerous side effects *and can only work when patients take them exactly as prescribed,* which is highly unlikely outside the sort of institutional setting that is no longer available. Yet government does not learn from its mistakes—and often refuses even to acknowledge that they *are* mistakes.

That is how the well-meaning but severely flawed program of deinstitutionalization connects to the well-meaning but severely flawed program of fighting prescription drug abuse. The development of ever-more-effective pain medications to relieve the suffering of tens of millions of people has led to a subculture of abuse by a small minority—resulting in government laws aimed at that minority but having the unintended consequence of severely damaging the lives of a vast number of law-abiding citizens. And the government has trod this exact road before, and not long ago—by making it much harder for law-abiding citizens to buy cold medicines containing the very effective decongestant *pseudoephedrine*.

3

Attack on Pseudoephedrine

Pseudoephedrine is best known for its decongestant effect—shrinking swollen nasal mucous membranes. It is quite effective for people with colds or allergies, increasing sinus drainage and helping open clogged Eustachian tubes. Pseudoephedrine has long been an ingredient of choice for symptomatic relief of cold and allergy symptoms. It is inexpensive and has few side effects unless used in excessive dosages or for a long time—when, like other stimulants, it can cause hypertension, sweating, insomnia and anxiety. Why then did the government take enforcement action against pseudoephedrine, even though it had been in use for nearly a century?

Attempts to control sales of pseudoephedrine date back to the mid-1980s, when the Drug Enforcement Administration tried to place numerous chemicals that could be used to make illicit recreational drugs under the Controlled Substances Act. Doing that required a new law, so the DEA wrote one. The DEA's plan would have required each transaction involving pseudoephedrine to be reported to the government and would have required federal approval of all imports and exports—thereby severely limiting legitimate pseudoephedrine use. Nice try, but it didn't work: after lobbying by manufacturers of over-the-counter medicines, chemicals that had been turned into legal final products, such as cold-symptom remedies, were exempted from the regulations.

What the DEA Did

THE DEA WAS PATIENT AND PERSISTENT, however. Undaunted, it kept pushing for strong regulation of pseudoephedrine and other chemicals that—while not dangerous in themselves—might be used to make illegal drugs. If this sounds like what later happened—and continues to happen—with opioid pain medication, it should, because it is the same approach. The DEA continues to clamp down on useful, legal medicines—at considerable inconvenience and potential danger to law-abiding citizens who need them—to curtail the small number of people who might misuse them.

The DEA eventually got what it wanted when Congress, in amending the USA PATRIOT Act, passed the *Combat Methamphetamine Epidemic Act of 2005* (CMEA). CMEA created a host of regulations affecting not only pseudoephedrine but also ephedrine and phenylpropanolamine and these compounds' salts, optical isomers, and salts of optical isomers. CMEA imposed the following mandates on sale of these popular, beneficial chemicals.

CMEA Mandate

Required a retrievable record of all purchases, identifying the name and address of each party, to be kept for two years.

Required verification of proof of identity of all purchasers.

Required protection and disclosure methods in the collection of personal information.

Required reports to the United States Attorney General of any suspicious payments or disappearances of the regulated products.

Required training of employees with regard to the requirements of the CMEA, with retailers self-certifying acceptable-to-the-government training and compliance.

The non-liquid-dose form of regulated products (pills, capsules & gelcaps) could only be sold in unit-dose blister packs

Regulated products were required to be stored behind the counter or in a locked cabinet in such a way as to restrict public access.

Sales Limits Per Customer

Daily sales limit: must not exceed 3.6 grams of pseudoephedrine base without regard to the number of transactions.

30-day—not monthly—sales limit: must not exceed 7.5 grams of pseudoephedrine base if sold by mail order or "mobile retail vendor."

30-day purchase limit: must not exceed 9 grams of pseudoephedrine base. The *buyer* who obtained more than this amount would be found guilty of misdemeanor possession of a controlled substance.

Acceptable Proof

WHILE THIS MAY SEEM LIKE OVERKILL to someone with a bad cold, to the DEA these restrictions are perfectly reasonable. In fact, CMEA went so far as to specify what "verification of proof of identity of all purchasers" merchants would be allowed to accept.

Verification of Identity

U.S. passport

U.S. military card

School ID with picture

Voter registration card

Native American tribal document

Alien registration or permanent
resident card

Unexpired foreign passport with
temporary I-551 stamp

Unexpired Employment
Authorization Document

Driver's license or government-
issued identification card, including
Canadian driver's license

Most states came up with their own laws paralleling
CMEA; Ohio's—sections 2925.55 to 2925.58 of the
Revised Code—is typical. It is painful to read both because of the tremendously overblown language in which
it is written and because of its content. Here is a very,
very small excerpt from the Revised Code.

Ohio Bows to CMEA

*(B)(1) No individual shall knowingly purchase,
receive, or otherwise acquire more than nine grams
of any pseudoephedrine product within a period of
thirty consecutive days, unless the pseudoephedrine
product is dispensed by a pharmacist pursuant to a
valid prescription issued by a licensed health professional authorized to prescribe drugs and the conduct*

*of the pharmacist and the licensed health professional
authorized to prescribe drugs is in accordance with
Chapter 3719, 4715, 4723, 4729, 4731, or 4741
of the Revised Code. ...*

*(C)(1) No individual under eighteen years of age
shall knowingly purchase, receive, or otherwise
acquire a pseudoephedrine product, unless the pseudoephedrine product is dispensed by a pharmacist
pursuant to a valid prescription issued by a licensed
health professional authorized to prescribe drugs and
the conduct of the pharmacist and the licensed health
professional authorized to prescribe drugs is in accordance with Chapter 3719, 4715, 4723, 4729, 4731,
or 4741 of the Revised Code.*

There is much more. Oh—and violations of the pro-
visions of Ohio's law are misdemeanors of the first or
fourth degree, depending on exactly what is violated
under exactly which circumstances.

The phrase "dangerous drugs" appears repeatedly
throughout Ohio's law, reflecting the DEA's determi-
nation to place pseudoephedrine and other substances in the category of dangerous

*Pseudoephedrine and the other
drugs covered by this statute have
been legally placed in the category of
dangerous drugs even though they
are not dangerous.*

drugs *even though they are not dangerous.* Yes, an underground chemist can convert pseudoephedrine into
methamphetamine, which *is* dangerous, but pseudoephedrine itself is not.

Planned Inconvenience

IT IS DEBATABLE whether this language is an intended or unintended consequence. What is *not* debatable is that CMEA and the state laws based on it created a complicated set of reporting requirements for pharmacists, making it highly inconvenient for people with colds or allergies to get the remedies they needed and had used for years without any problems. For example, these products could only be sold during hours when pharmacists were on duty and able to record the purchase. Anyone needing medicine in the middle of the night, or on a weekend, would just have to go without.

One reason the crackdown on pseudoephedrine failed to raise a public outcry was that there had been widespread reporting of the dangers of methamphetamine. Additionally, manufacturers had a super-

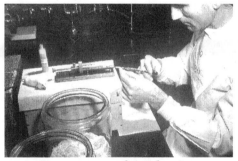

Drug research with mice

ficially similar ingredient available—phenylephrine, whose name even sounds similar to pseudoephedrine. Drug makers made it appear that a seamless transition to phenylephrine—an equally good medicine—was simple. They even made up new brand names close to those of popular pseudoephedrine-containing products. Sudafed® contains pseudoephedrine, while Sudafed PE® contains phenylephrine instead, for example.

Imposing a Limit

IT TAKES RESEARCH to find out the amounts of chemicals that are effective and those that are dangerous. But laws simply impose a limit—often an arbitrary one. The government actually felt it was doing people a favor by not requiring all sales of pseudoephedrine-containing products to be by prescription only—as prescriptions were already required for alternative decongestant products such as Nasonex® and Flonase®. Those are steroid-based nasal inhalants that, like products containing pseudoephedrine, reduce swelling in the sinuses. But the steroid inhalants cost considerably more than products containing pseudoephedrine, require a doctor's visit to get a prescription, and take several days to work, while products that include pseudoephedrine require no prescription and work quickly.

*D*rug makers went out of their way to make it appear that a seamless transition to an equally good medicine was simple.

So why not simply switch to products that use phenylephrine? The answer is simple: for many people, they do not work—certainly not as well as those containing pseudoephedrine.

Inconvenience for all is the collateral damage of the attack on pseudoephedrine—inconvenience for sellers of effective over-the-counter congestion-relieving products, inconvenience for buyers unable to get the products when they need them, and inconvenience and expense for patients having to go to the doctor to get a prescription for more-expensive alternative medicine.

Intended Consequences

IT IS ARGUABLE whether these effects should be called "unintended" consequences, since there is much to suggest that the DEA *intended* to make it harder for honest people to dispense and obtain pseudoephedrine products in order to prevent a small number of criminals from misusing them. Because cold and allergy symptoms are acute rather than chronic and are generally comparatively mild, and some alternatives to pseudoephedrine-containing products do exist,

For many people, products containing phenylephrine do not work.

the argument could be—and was—made that relatively minor inconveniences for a very large number of people did not matter, compared to the goal of preventing the manufacture of methamphetamine. But these rules have *not* prevented underground chemists from continuing to cook up meth—yet similar arguments are being used to make it harder for pain patients to obtain opioids.

4

Government on Opioids

The U.S. government as a whole is more concerned about prescription-drug abuse than about making sure the people who need legal dugs receive them in a timely and effective manner. And it is easy to understand why the parts of the government charged with developing and enforcing anti-drug policies feel this way. But the government is huge and not monolithic, and it is not so easy to understand why the Centers for Disease Control and Prevention (CDC)—the medical division of the government—merely pays lip service to the value of drugs that control pain, then quickly starts to talk about limiting use of those drugs because of the possibility of their abuse by a small minority of people.

Nevertheless, that is what the CDC does. There is no single overarching document setting forth CDC policy in this area, as there is from the Office of National Drug Control Policy (see Chapter 5). But through presentations to the media and fellow researchers, and in highly respected publications such as *Morbidity and Mortality Weekly Report* or MMWR, doctors and others at the CDC have presented an overview of CDC thinking about prescription drug abuse.

One prominent doctor, Leonard Paulozzi, MD, of the CDC's Division of Unintentional Injury Prevention—part of the National Center for Injury Prevention and Control—has written, with six coauthors, that prescription drug abuse was the fastest-growing drug problem in the United States in the early 21st century, noting that between 2003 and 2012, more overdose deaths involved opioid analgesics than heroin and cocaine combined. And the problem was described as even bigger than that: for every unintentional overdose death related to an opioid analgesic, nine people require substance-abuse treatment, 35 visit emergency departments, and 161 report drug abuse or dependence.

So from the CDC viewpoint, yes, there is certainly a prescription-drug-overdose problem; and yes, it is societal as well as personal; and yes, it makes sense for medical professionals to pay attention to it and be concerned about it. The CDC doctors' focus is primarily on opioids and on those who abuse them— but "abuse" is never precisely defined.

Prescription drug abuse is the fastest growing drug problem in the United States.

–Centers for Disease Control and Prevention

And this is where things get muddy. Under government thinking, *any* misuse of a prescription drug may be deemed "abuse." Someone who is prescribed a drug for an illness, keeps some that is left over after the illness runs its course, and later takes it for a different illness, is officially an abuser. That is "government think." But most people would define "abuse" differently, associating it with deliberate use of prescription medicines recreationally. The distinction matters—because what the government seeks to control, and what concerns the CDC, is much broader than what disturbs most people.

Identifying Drug Abusers

ACCORDING TO DR. PAULOZZI and his coauthors, each month about nine million people report long-term medical use of opioids, and about five million use them without a prescription or medical need. The five million are the ones most people would think of as drug abusers. To the government, though, the nine million people with chronic pain—a medical need for pain relief—are almost twice as likely as thrill-seekers to abuse drugs and overdose. Few people outside government would think of this as prescription drug abuse, however. Most would understand that someone with severe pain may take an extra dose of medicine to try to relieve the agony, and that is abuse only in the narrowest and most legalistic of senses.

The CDC doctors admit that MDs can find themselves in a difficult position when taking care of patients. Because opioids are so effective against pain, doctors have been prescribing more and more of them. As a result, "Persons who abuse opioids have learned to exploit this new practitioner sensitivity to patient pain, and clinicians struggle to treat patients without over-prescribing these drugs."

The CDC doctors' breakdown of the types of patients for whom opioids are typically prescribed produces some interesting statistics. An estimated 80% of patients are prescribed low opioid doses by a single practitioner—and those patients account for about 20% of all prescription drug overdoses. Another 10% of patients are prescribed high doses by single prescribers, and account

Persons who abuse opioids have learned to exploit this new practitioner sensitivity to patient pain.

–Leonard Paulozzi, M.D.

for an estimated 40% of prescription opioid overdoses. And the final 10% do "doctor shopping," seeking care from multiple doctors and ending up with high daily doses. The people in this last group "not only are at high risk for overdose themselves but are likely

The CDC article falls back on the same strategy that the DEA pursues: restrict and clamp down.

diverting or providing drugs to others who are using them without prescriptions." That is, they are not only abusers but also enablers of others' abuse.

The 80-20 Rule

THE STATISTICS ARE IN LINE with the Pareto principle, more commonly known as the 80-20 rule, which indicates that roughly 80% of effects come from roughly 20% of causes. Here we see that 80% of patients with opioid prescriptions receive low doses, and those patients account for only 20% of overdoses—while 20% of patients receive high doses and account for 80% of the overdose problem. Clearly a concerted, effective effort to deal with opioid overuse or abuse needs to focus on the 20% of people responsible for 80% of the problem, and not limit the ability of 80% of patients to obtain and use the medications they need. It would be reasonable to expect the CDC to call for this.

But this is not what the CDC does, and its doctors do not address patient needs head-on. Instead, they fall back on the same strategy the Drug Enforcement Administration pursues—restrict and clamp down on drug supplies in general. Specifically, the doctors make three suggestions for dealing with opioid overdose and abuse, the first two of which could just as easily have been written by the DEA as by the CDC:

CDC Recommendations

Integrate prescription information with insurance restrictions to prevent "doctor shopping." Track people through state databases and insurance claims. Limit reimbursement of claims for opioid prescriptions to a single designated doctor and single designated pharmacy for each patient.

Strictly enforce existing punitive laws, pass more of them, and get states to pass stronger laws and enforce them uniformly.

Change the practice of medicine as it relates to pain amelioration. Create guidelines for opioid use in regular medical practices and in hospital emergency departments—and have "health system or payer reviews hold prescribers accountable for their behaviors."

That last sentence is particularly significant, arguing that "payer reviews"—that is, reviews by insurance companies and government insurance programs— should be used to hold doctors accountable for their medical decisions regarding the use of opioids. This would be a major intrusion into the doctor-patient relationship. So would the first recommendation, which would encourage insurers, both governmental and private-sector, to "identify inappropriate use of certain opioids for certain diagnoses." Coming from the CDC's medical professionals, these are extremely disturbing recommendations, urging greater involvement by government officials and insurance companies in everyday decision-making about treatment of severe pain.

The CDC doctors do not practice patient-focused medicine for a living—they are government employees—but they do have medical training. The fact that they recommend this level of government intrusion into the doctor-patient relationship is extremely troubling—and unfortunately typical of government overreaching in the name of preventing abuse by a small minority.

Insurance companies and the government would hold doctors accountable for their medical decisions.

Lack of Alternatives

A REASONABLE QUESTION to ask is what the CDC would have doctors do instead of prescribing an opioid. The CDC doctors do not assert that most such prescriptions are for unusually high doses of medicine—remember the comment that "80% of patients with opioid prescriptions receive low doses from a single prescriber." They are therefore not making a recommendation to prescribe opioids carefully but are in effect offering a proposal to cut back on using them at all. And do what instead? On that topic, the CDC is as silent as the DEA. But surely the CDC's medical doctors are aware that there are *no* medicines as effective as opioids currently available for the purposes for which opioids are generally—80% of the time—prescribed properly and appropriately.

There are no medicines as effective as opioids currently available for the purposes for which opioids are generally prescribed.

The CDC doctors single out certain states for praise for their legal and regulatory efforts to deal with opioid overdose or abuse, but say clearly that a state-by-state approach is not enough—something must be done uniformly, at the federal level. And again they make a passing reference, but only a passing one, to the crucial issue of making sure that patients in severe, chronic pain have access to the only medicines that can give them even a modicum of quality of life. "When developing a national approach to address prescription drug overdose, any policy must balance the desire to minimize abuse with the need to ensure legitimate access to these medications, and its implementation must bring together a variety of federal, state, local, and tribal groups."

Specifically, the CDC endorses a four-part plan developed under the auspices of the White House Office of National Drug Control Policy and the DEA. And this is a very troubling position, because that plan— the primary government response to prescription-drug abuse—specifically *omits* any discussion of the importance of caring for patients with severe, chronic pain.

5

Government Responds

Always read the footnotes first. This is excellent advice when examining financial documents and trying to decide, for example, whether or not to invest in a company's stock. It is also solid advice when it comes to government documents. "The devil is in the detail," the saying goes, and there is nothing more detailed, or sometimes devilish, than the footnotes to a government report.

The government document guiding the official response to prescription drug abuse, released by the White House with considerable fanfare, is an eleven-page report by the Office of National Drug Control Policy, ONDCP, outlining steps to deal with abuse of medicines. The report, somewhat melodramatically entitled *Epidemic: Responding to America's Prescription Drug Abuse Crisis,* includes twenty footnotes, most referring to data sources used in its preparation. The footnote to read carefully is the very last one, which is quite short: "Accomplishment of the plan and its goals is dependent on the availability of resources." Translation: the government says it knows what to do about prescription drug abuse as long as the funding, staffing and other forms of commitment are there.

Leaving aside the question of whether this final footnote, at the bottom of the report's last page, renders the whole exercise moot, it is worth exploring what the government "knows" can be done to deal with what the report calls "the Nation's fastest-growing drug problem."

Extent of the Problem

THE IMPORTANT THING to understand about government documents in the United States is that they are not written in English as most of us understand the language. Our lawmakers are, by and large, lawyers, and while the Founding Fathers—who, by and large, were *not* lawyers—wrote astonishingly memorable and understandable prose, their modern successors are mostly concerned with dotting the i's and crossing the t's in convoluted legal-speak—while readers cross *their* eyes with confusion.

Much of the clearest writing from ONDCP comes in simple recitation of statistics, and those statistics do show the extent of the prescription-drug-abuse problem: "From 1997 to 2007, the milligram per person use of prescription opioids in the U.S. increased from 74 milligrams to 369 milligrams, an increase of 402 percent. In addition, in 2000, retail pharmacies dispensed 174 million prescriptions for opioids; by 2009, 257 million prescriptions were dispensed, an increase of 48 percent." Dealing with prescription drug abuse, the ONDCP says—in a passage whose call for common effort recurs throughout its document—requires involvement by parents, patients, healthcare providers, and manufacturers.

The primary problem of opioid abuse does not lie with the medical profession.

Opioid abuse cuts across all segments of society, the report says, noting—correctly—that the primary problem does not lie with the medical profession. More than seventy percent of people who abused prescription pain relievers got them from friends or relatives, compared with just five percent who got them from a drug dealer or from the Internet. *O*ver 70 percent of people who Citing the abused prescription pain relievers Monitoring got them from friends or relatives. the Future —Government survey study—the nation's largest survey of drug use among young people—the ONDCP said that prescription drugs are the second-most-abused category of drugs after marijuana, and that in the armed forces, illicit drug use went up from five percent to twelve percent within a single three-year period, from 2005 to 2008, mainly because of prescription drug abuse.

As usual in government documents, lip service is paid to the importance of opioids for control of chronic, severe pain: "The potent medications science has developed have great potential for relieving suffering, as well as great potential for abuse. ...Accordingly, any policy in this area must strike a balance between our desire to minimize abuse of prescription drugs and the need to ensure access for their legitimate use."

Drug Control Above All

HOWEVER, the report immediately goes on to say that its recommendations are based on the National Drug Control Strategy; and there is no further attention paid to the enormous and undoubted benefits of pain-relief medications. Instead there is the outline of a four-part approach to prescription drug abuse. ONDCP says that, first, education is critical to boost awareness of the dangers of prescription drug abuse. Second, "enhancement and increased utilization of prescription drug monitoring programs will help to identify 'doctor shoppers' and detect therapeutic duplication and drug-drug interactions," which in everyday English means more closely watching doctors and pharmacists to try to get a handle on patients who get multiple prescriptions by going from one medical office to the next to the one after that.

The ONDCP's third focus is on "consumer-friendly and environmentally-responsible prescription drug disposal programs," the idea being to make it harder for abusers to get drugs from family members and friends—as most do. And the fourth focus is on giving law-enforcement agencies "the tools they need" to shut down doctor shopping and drug overuse—a prescription so broadly stated that it inherently contains abuse potential of its own.

Although these four elements sound reasonable enough when stated simplistically, the devil remains in the detail, and it is worth looking at each of the four in more detail to see what the government thinks it can do—and whether its proposals are realistic and sensitive to the very real needs of patients who endure chronic, excruciating pain day in and day out.

Education

THE ONDCP SAYS many people remain unaware that the abuse of prescription drugs can be as dangerous as the use of illegal drugs, pointing to the common misperception that prescription drugs are less dangerous when abused than illegal drugs because they are approved for medical use by the Food and Drug Administration. The report says parents are unaware of the risks of giving drugs to family members for whom they were not prescribed—and sometimes entirely unaware that young people abuse prescription medicines. Therefore, many parents "frequently leave unused prescription drugs in open medicine cabinets while making sure to lock their liquor cabinets."

This may be true, but it seems to be irrelevant. Studies of child poisonings by the nonprofit organization Safe Kids Worldwide have found that most kids get medicines from older *Medicine misuse often results from bottles dropped on the floor or otherwise misplaced.* adults—usually mothers and grandmothers—who leave them in purses or pillboxes or out on counters, for easy access and to help themselves remember to take multiple pills. And more than one-quarter of medicines misused by children come from bottles dropped on the floor or otherwise misplaced. There is no reason to suspect a significantly different pattern for medications misused by older children or teenagers.

Curiously, ONDCP does not say that medicine cabinets should start coming with strong locks. But it does spread some blame beyond the family by criticizing drug manufacturers' direct-to-consumer advertising for contributing to higher demand for medicines—although it is a little bit difficult to see just what in the advertising makes the drugs so attractive to anybody, including those who really need them, given the sorts of conditions for which manufacturers advertise their medications and the extent of the disclaimers they include in the ads.

So we have finger-pointing at 1) parents; 2) teenagers and other young people; 3) drug manufacturers for their advertising; and 4) the media that transmit the ads. The ONDCP says the combination of these factors makes education against prescription drug abuse all the more important. Nor are these the only bad guys in the ONDCP's worldview:

The government points the finger of blame at parents, teenagers, drug manufacturers and the media.

"Prescribers and dispensers, including physicians, physicians assistants, nurse practitioners, pharmacists, nurses, prescribing psychologists, and dentists, all have a role to play in reducing prescription drug misuse and abuse. Most receive little training on the importance of appropriate prescribing and dispensing of opioids to prevent adverse effects, diversion, and addiction."

Indeed, it is not only members of the health-care profession who are at fault, the report says—so are the places where they get their training, because most medical, dental, pharmacy, and other schools for healthcare professionals do not provide in-depth training on substance abuse or, for that matter, on pain treatment. So the ONDCP maintains.

So now it is time for action items, and there are thirteen of them, in three areas designated "Healthcare Provider Education," "Parent, Youth, and Patient Education," and "Research and Development." And here some of those devils of detail raise their heads. ONDCP works from an underlying assumption that cross-agency cooperation within the federal government is a norm or is easily attainable for an issue of national significance, such as prescription drug abuse. Does anyone outside the federal government believe this? Does anyone *inside* the government *really* believe it? The problem from the start is that action items that sound reasonable on their face require, for implementation, a level of interagency coordination that is entirely out of the question—witness the many reports, dating back many years, of agencies tripping over their own feet and those of other agencies while trying to get something done.

In the matter of healthcare provider education, for instance, ONDCP reasonably talks about working to encourage the overseers of schools for health professionals—medical, dental, nursing and pharmacy—to spend more time in classes instructing students on better use of opioids. This also includes working with student groups to establish programs that would give community educational presentations on prescription drug abuse and substance abuse. Not a bad concept. But how would it be done? ONDCP says it requires a veritable alphabet soup of federal agencies to work together: HHS, SAMHSA, ONDCP, FDA, HRSA, NIDA, DOD and VA.

Extensive Coordination

IN ORDINARY ENGLISH, that means this idea alone requires coordination among the Department of Health and Human Services, the Substance Abuse and Mental Health Services Administration, the White House Office of National Drug Control Policy, the Food and Drug Administration, the Health Resources and Ser-

Does anyone really believe that cross-agency cooperation within the federal government is a norm or is easily attainable?

vices Administration, the National Institute on Drug Abuse, the Department of Defense, and the Veterans Administration. Remember that footnote number 20? Does anyone really believe that this idea, even if it is a good one, will ever come close to implementation?

Apparently the answer is yes, since there are twelve more like it. In just one more example, from the "Parent, Youth, and Patient Education" section, ONDCP urges "all stakeholders" to "support and promote an evidence-based public education campaign" about the right way to use, store and dispose of prescription drugs. This would involve local anti-drug coalitions, chain pharmacies, community pharmacies, boards of pharmacies, boards of medicine and other groups in raising awareness of prescription drug misuse and abuse. The federal participants? That would be ONDCP, CDC, FDA, DEA, IHS, ED, SAMHSA, DOD, VA and EPA.

Yes, this recommendation adds the Centers for Disease Control and Prevention, the Drug Enforcement Administration, the Indian Health Service, the Education Department, and the Environmental Protection Agency to the mix of federal groups expected to act together. The coordination involved, given the way government bureaucracies function, is out of the question, quite apart from footnote number 20, which throws all the planning into limbo. As a statement of ideals, this portion of the *Epidemic* document is more meaningful than as a plan that is ever likely to be implemented. But how about other portions of the report?

Tracking and Monitoring

THIS SECTION OPENS WITH a note that forty-three states have authorized prescription drug monitoring programs, known as PDMPs, whose aim is to detect and prevent the diversion and abuse of prescription drugs at the retail level, and make it easier to collect and analyze prescription data more efficiently. Of the forty-three, though, ONDCP points out that just thirty-five actually have working PDMPs, which have to be authorized by state legislation and then paid for by a combination of state and federal funds.

The report says PDMPs are useful in reducing drug diversion, but may not be operating at maximum effective-ness, so additional work is needed to make them more

Again, substantial coordination is assumed with all the states and among, in this case, seven federal agencies.

effective. And to do that, once again, substantial coordi-nation is assumed with all the states and among, in this case, seven federal agencies: ONDCP, SAMHSA, NIDA, CDC and three not mentioned before—the Department of Justice, National Institute of Justice, and Office of the National Coordinator for Health Information.

It should be apparent by this point that the entire *Epidemic* report assumes a level of cooperation among federal agencies and between government at the federal and state levels beyond anything that has occurred in the past or could reasonably be expected to happen in the future, even if sufficient funding were to be made available—which, in light of footnote number 20, is clearly not to be expected. Every idea presented in the report, whether compulsory or advisory, is similar in this regard. What happens is that the issue of patient care, never in the forefront of government thinking about medication use, essentially disappears altogether, being supplanted by a series of suggestions—reasonable on the surface—that in practice would be extremely difficult, if not impossible, to implement, and that exist within an environment in which the primary concern is *not* patient care but the creation of elaborate systems to deal with the misuse of drugs that, when used properly, are crucial to patient health.

And the financial issue keeps coming up as well: "We must identify stable financial support to maximize the utility of PDMPs, which will help reduce prescription drug diversion and provide better healthcare delivery"—as if the only problem lies in *identifying* this sort of "stable financial support" for the recommendations. The implication is that such financial support does exist; it is only a matter of finding it.

It would be unfair to argue that the ONDCP ideas for education and for tracking and monitoring are ill-motivated, or that the creators of the *Epidemic* report do not themselves believe in the plan. Certainly Gil Kerlikowske, director of ONDCP, sounded sincere when he said that the plan provides a national framework, on a collaborative basis, for reducing prescription drug abuse and the diversion of prescription drugs for recreational use.

Suggestions that seem reasonable on the surface would in practice be extremely difficult, if not impossible, to implement.

"The toll our nation's prescription drug abuse epidemic has taken in communities nationwide is devastating," said Kerlikowske. "We share a responsibility to protect our communities from the damage done by prescription drug abuse." But moving from shared responsibility to cooperative action is a very tall order, if it is possible at all. This issue not only affects the question of whether the educational and tracking-and-monitoring proposals are doable, but also is relevant to the report's recommendations on medication disposal—and enforcement.

6

Disposal & Enforcement

The official federal government response to the problem of prescription drug abuse, known as *Epidemic: Responding to America's Prescription Drug Abuse Crisis*, goes beyond educational and tracking-and-monitoring recommendations. It says there are two other elements needed to deal with abuse of the medicines: proper disposal and, quite emphatically, law enforcement—which lies at the heart of all government programs against illicit drugs and against misuse of legal ones.

Proper Medication Disposal

WE HAVE ALL DONE IT: used some but not all of a prescription and then left the remainder in a medicine cabinet or tossed it in a drawer somewhere. Medicines are expensive, and there is always the chance that we may need one again even though we no longer need it at a given time. After a dental procedure, for example, a painkiller of some sort may be prescribed, but if the pain is not as great as expected or we simply do not want to take more medicine than absolutely necessary, we may find we have some left. In fact, if the dentist— or doctor or other health-care practitioner—has done a good job explaining concerns about opioids, we may be less likely to use everything prescribed.

But everyone has unexpected, acute pain now and then—a severely sprained ankle, perhaps, or a muscle spasm, an abrasion from a fall, back pain from lifting something heavy, and so on—so why not hold onto any leftover medicine just in case we might need it in the future? Even if medicine is past its expiration date, it will still have *some* effect, and it just seems to make sense to keep it on hand in case of a future need. After all, it was prescribed once—and what if we have an injury at a time when we cannot get to a doctor, such as at night or on a weekend or holiday? What if we know the injury does not merit a doctor's appointment but is still very painful? Better to have something around just in case.

Even if medicine is past its expiration date, it will still have some effect, and it just seems to make sense to keep it on hand in case of a future need.

This is perfectly reasonable thinking, but the ONDCP report wants it changed where opioids are concerned, because "a large source of the problem [of prescription drug abuse] is a direct result of what is in Americans' medicine cabinets." So the government wants a focus on getting rid of unused medicines in a secure and convenient way—with the side benefit, ONDCP notes, of reducing the introduction of drugs into the environment.

Other Government Concerns

THE *EPIDEMIC* REPORT TOUCHES ON other, more-general concerns of the federal government. For instance, it

acknowledges that drug disposal must be done in accord
with laws and regulations at all levels—federal, state and
local. And it urges widespread dissemination of a message
telling people not to flush prescription drugs—except
that it is all right to flush *some* of them, according to the
Food and Drug Administration. So how should people
dispose of medicines? Simple, says the report: in sealed
plastic bags with filler such as coffee grounds or kitty litter. Unless, of course, we are talking about certain opioid
pain relievers, which could pose life-threatening risks if
taken accidentally. Those *should* be flushed.

Simple? This whole portion of the report is a bit off-
topic and a bit confusing, since it deals first with environmental issues, than suggests a form of disposal that
very, very few individuals are ever likely to use—putting the medicine in sealed plastic bags and adding used
coffee grounds or kitty litter—and then says that flush-
ing actually *is* recommended for *certain* opioids, without
specifying which ones. As a result of this imprecision,
the three recommended actions in this section of the
Epidemic report are, not surprisingly, weak. They involve distributing information on "take-back activities," educating the public about new regulations on
drug disposal when such regulations are established, and
urging the private sector to support community-based
medication disposal programs.

Enforcement

BUT IF THE RECOMMENDATIONS on disposal are weak,
those on enforcment are strong. This is, after all, the
area where the government commits the vast majority
of its anti-drug efforts: interdiction. The report comes
down hard on "a small group of practitioners who abuse
their prescribing privileges by prescribing these medica-

tions outside the usual course of professional practice or for illegitimate purposes." This small group endangers individuals and the community, the report says. And there is also the problem of doctor shopping, in which abusers visit multiple prescribers in their own states and others, to get medications that they then abuse or pass along to others.

Enforcement is the area where the government commits the vast majority of its anti-drug efforts.

Dealing with these issues, says the report, requires community based-solutions.

But community-based solutions are not within the purview of the federal government. The *Epidemic* report nevertheless makes eight recommendations for action here, all in the context of assisting states in dealing with problems.

Some Government Plans

AGGRESSIVE ENFORCEMENT action against pain clinics and prescribers that abuse their right to prescribe medication.

Greater intelligence-gathering and investigation of prescription drug trafficking, including an increase in the number of joint investigations by federal, state, and local agencies.

Expansion of the Prescription Drug Monitoring Program so its data can be used to identify criminal prescribers and clinics by the volume of selected drugs prescribed.

It is in these enforcement areas that federal recommendations are really strong—and themselves really subject to abuse. The third idea above, for example, through its focus on "the volume of selected drugs prescribed," is an obvious example of potential damage to doctors and clinics specifically set up and maintained to mitigate severe, chronic pain. Safeguards against abuse by authorities would theoretically be established—although they are nowhere mentioned in the *Epidemic* report—but it is easy to see how this sort of crackdown would have a chilling effect on practitioners and clinics whose focus is pain mitigation.

To some extent, such an effect is inevitable. Just as Willy Sutton famously said that he robbed banks because "that's where the money is," abuse of opioids is more likely to occur in places where lots of them are prescribed and used, because that's where the drugs are. But this is precisely where the issue of treating chronic, debilitating pain comes into conflict with that of preventing abuse of the medications used to control pain and make sufferers' lives bearable. The human element, the patient element, is entirely missing from the *Epidemic* report, which refers to people's suffering only in passing and only in bland bureaucratese.

The *Epidemic* report concludes with a series of goals, the first of which is a five-year goal presented in classic governmentalese: a "15 percent reduction in non-medical use of prescription-type psychotherapeutic drugs in the past year

The government report refers to people's suffering only in passing and only in bland bureaucratese.

among people 12 years of age and older." Compared to everyday English, the language is confusing: what it means is that abuse statistics are based on reported misuse of drugs during the past year—so the stated goal is, by 2016, to have fifteen percent fewer reports of such misuse. But this is a peculiar recommendation, because it deals with *psychotherapeutic* drugs, not opioids, and the entire remainder of the *Epidemic* report focuses on opioid abuse. It is almost as if some of the preparers of the *Epidemic* report lost focus when creating this recommendation—or realized, belatedly, that psychotherapeutics as well as opioids can be abused by some people under some circumstances. Regardless of the reason for the appearance of this goal, it is not followed up—all remaining elements of the *Epidemic* report return to a focus on opioids.

Thirteen Further Elements

AND THERE ARE THIRTEEN additional elements, gathered under the heading "Prescription Drug Abuse Prevention Plan Goals." These goals range from working with "stakeholders" on public education about opioids, to getting legislation passed requiring health professionals to have specific training on opioid use and misuse, to getting a number of federal agencies—including the Department of Defense, Veterans Administration and Indian Health Service—to provide prescription information electronically to Prescription Drug Monitoring Programs in states in which they operate healthcare facilities and pharmacies. Another goal is to have legislation in all fifty states establishing PDMPs, and another is to expand by ten percent the amount of funding for treatment of drug abusers, only a small percentage of whom currently obtain treatment.

To say that these plans are highly optimistic is an understatement. They require coordination among multiple federal agencies, cooperation with the legislatures in all fifty states, the drafting and passage of federal legislation, and increased funding for a particular purpose. A ten percent increase may not seem like much, but additional funding for drug treatment—as opposed to drug interdiction—has been a hard sell for many years.

The ultimate objective here is unexceptionable and certainly well-meaning: "Decrease by 15 percent the number of unintentional overdose deaths related to opioids within 60 months." It is hard to imagine any politician or any appointed or elected bureaucrat objecting to this, and in fact it is easy to imagine members of the government insisting that a fifteen percent reduction in deaths is too modest a goal. But

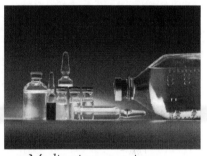

Medication containers

that would be grandstanding in the absence of backing for the various initiatives elsewhere in the *Epidemic* report—and absence of the interagency cooperation and funding needed to implement them. Since neither cooperation across so many agencies nor permanent funding at the levels needed can be deemed at all likely, it is fair to assess the entire *Epidemic* report itself as a form of grandstanding—well-meaning grandstanding, but grandstanding nevertheless.

No one is likely to argue against the report's summary comment: "As a Nation, we must take urgent action to ensure the appropriate balance between the benefits these medications offer in improving lives and the risks they pose." But getting to that balance is not as straightforward as the report indicates; and indeed, the patient-care component, the one focusing on benefits, is notably absent from the report, except in passing and in mild language that in effect pays lip service to the good done by pain-relief drugs while focusing far more on their dangers.

It is clear that the government does *not* focus on the patients who really need these medicines. The government—whether federal, state or local—does not practice medicine, so a lack of patient focus may seem inevitable. But the nature of government focus on abuse of pain medicines leads to significant restrictions on the doctor-patient relationship—in effect altering the practice of medicine by requiring that it be handled within limits that the government considers appropriate, not ones that medical professionals themselves deem correct. The result is an enormous amount of unnecessary suffering. And yes, it could happen to you—or to someone in your family.

Getting to a balance between the benefits of medications and the risks they pose is not as straightforward as the government indicates.

7

Victimizing the Victims

The government knows one and only one way to mark success in its war on prescription drug abuse—with the equivalent of a body count in other kinds of war. For example, in June 2012, the Drug Enforcement Administration was proud to announce that it had broken an operation in South Florida that had bought 19,000 oxycodone pills in one year, intending to resell them.

But this is not the real body count, not in Florida and not nationally. The real body count includes a Florida nurse whose car was rear-ended by a truck as she was on the way to work; who needed spinal surgery for her injuries; who has had chronic pain ever since and can barely walk without medication; and who suddenly found herself unable to get pain medicines because the DEA deems pain patients to be the same sort of "collateral damage" that the government euphemistically talks about when innocent civilians are killed in wars. "I'm so tired of fighting every month so that I can have a life. It's unbearable anymore. I'm to the point where I just want to leave this stupid state because I'm tired of being treated like a drug addict when I've done

I'm so tired of fighting every month so that I can have a life.

–Patient with chronic pain

nothing wrong," the nurse told a Florida public broadcasting station in describing the extreme difficulty she was having in getting legitimate prescriptions for desperately needed pain medicine filled.

The body count also includes Christine Link, a Washington state resident who took prescription pain-killers for years because of a severe degenerative joint disease—until doctors, under government pressure, refused to refill her prescriptions. "I am suffering, and I know I am not the only one," Link told *The New York Times*.

A Pharmacist's Story

IN THE BODY COUNT as well are medication dispens-ers such as Mike Pavlovich, a pharmacist in Newport Beach, California, whose story was recounted by writer and chronic-pain sufferer Mark Maginn. Pavlovich's business suddenly stopped receiving its usual shipments of opioid medicines from its distributor. Why? Maginn found out that the DEA had accused Cardinal Health, Pavlovich's distributor, of supplying too many opioids to Florida pharmacies and not having adequate controls to detect diversion. So, after being heavily fined, Cardi-nal Health started checking the records of its pharmacy customers in other parts of the country—and decided that the number of prescriptions Pavlovich was filling for opioids and other controlled substances was too high for the company's comfort level.

But there was a good reason for the prescriptions: Pavlovich works with doctors who specialize in treating patients who suffer from chronic, debilitating pain; indeed, he was the only pharmacist on the U.S. Olympic Committee's medical team to travel to China for the Beijing Olympics in 2008. In fact, Pavlovich acts as a mentor, educating others on the safe filling of opioid prescriptions; and he told Maginn that he had never been cited by the State Board of Pharmacy or the DEA for any transgressions.

The DEA, however, did not and does not care. Maginn's article for *American News Report* explained that, no matter which large distributor Pavlovich contacted, none of them would fill his whole prescription order: "The DEA had cast a wide net. After further discussions he was able to secure only 15% of his oxycodone order from Cardinal Health."

By clamping down on Pavlovich's distributor, the DEA's actions did two things. First, the sudden major cutback in his drug stock risked crippling his business, affecting not only him and his family but also

Government actions harmed the business and gave some patients with debilitating pain nowhere to turn.

the families of his employees. Second, Pavlovich said it clearly affected patients who rely on opioids for pain control—after the reduction, Pavlovich was simply unable to fill legitimate prescriptions for many of his customers and had to turn a number of them away, leaving them to suffer. Maginn quoted Pavlovich as saying that the DEA's policy enforcement "has made it virtually impossible for a pharmacy that serves patients with chronic pain as their primary niche to meet the needs of its patients."

Lack of Information

PAVLOVICH TRIED TO FIND OUT exactly what level
of dispensing the DEA considers excessive. He was
not the only one to try—or the only one to fail. The
government is not obligated to help pharmacists fill
prescriptions for patients in desperate need of pain
relief—and it doesn't. Instead, it comes up with statistical, nonmedical formulas in which all pharmacies
are treated the same way, no matter what their patient
population may be and no matter how specialized they
may have become in handling the needs of patients in
severe, chronic pain. Pavlovich, for example, was told
that for every one hundred units or products sold, opioids might make up fifteen percent to forty percent of
sales volume—a very wide range that can be calculated
multiple ways, for example by quantity or dollar value—before the DEA would deem opioid sales excessive.

The DEA is not alone in its lack of concern for pain
patients. Its behavior is the most egregious of that of
any government agency, but that is because its mission is to restrict, confiscate and remove drugs from the
system, and its effectiveness is measured by how well
it does that. Sophisticated or merely careful and reasonable consideration of the legitimate needs of pain
patients takes time and effort, is outside the DEA's mandate, and does nothing to sustain and boost its funding.
So its actions are understandable in the context of how
government works.

Ideas from Congress

BUT THE DEA is abetted by the actions of others in
government—actions that are ideologically motivated.
California Rep. Mary Bono Mack, for example, intro-

duced in the 112th Congress a bill called the "Stop Oxy Abuse Act" that would mandate the use of oxycodone only for "severe" pain, not for "moderate-to-severe" pain—which was the Food and Drug Administration standard. Rep. Mack is not a doctor, has never treated a patient with chronic pain, and did not attempt to define the difference between "severe" and "moderate-to-severe" pain. In fact, as any medical student knows, one of the first lessons in

The bill would make it more difficult for doctors to practice medicine honestly.

medical school is that *pain is not an objective symptom.* Every individual who thinks about this is aware of it: we all know someone who seems to overreact to the smallest injury or headache, and someone else who seems to bear up under pain that we ourselves would consider unbearable. No matter—Rep. Mack wanted to legislate the indefinable.

And she introduced a second bill in the same Congress, designed to force doctors to get training or special certification—as approved not by medical authorities but by the Attorney General—in the "appropriate and safe use of controlled substances" such as pain medicines. What was particularly interesting about this attempt to force doctors to practice medicine as non-doctors choose to define it was that Rep. Mack called this bill the "Ryan Creedon Act," naming it after a twenty-one-year-old man from her district who died from an oxycodone overdose—*after he got the medicine by scamming doctors.* So by cheating and misleading doctors and taking medicines abusively and recreationally, thus ending his own life, Ryan Creedon got a proposed law named after him—a law intended *not* to weed out other Ryan Creedons but to make it more difficult for the doctors he scammed to practice medicine honestly.

No politician has yet proposed a Christine Link Act to benefit pain patients such as the Washington state resident. In fact, Washington state put itself at the epicenter of the pain-management vs. pain-abuse issue by stepping directly into the doctor-patient relationship in 2011, when its legislature *required* doctors not to allow patients to take medicine equivalent to more than one hundred twenty milligrams of morphine a day without referring them to a pain specialist. Why one hundred twenty milligrams? Because the legislators said so—without any input from doctors. Isn't that practicing medicine without a license?

8

Washington State's R_x

Luckily for them, legislators' oaths of office do not require them to swear that they will do no harm. To understand what the legislators in Washington state did, a trip back to 2006 is necessary. In that year, Gary M. Franklin, MD, MPH, research professor of environmental and occupational health sciences for the state, discovered that thirty-two workers treated under state worker-compensation law had died of opioid overdoses after being prescribed the drugs. He found that the strength of the average daily opioid dose prescribed to patients had increased fifty percent, while the number of patients taking the drugs at high doses had grown to ten thousand.

Dr. Franklin called a meeting of fifteen medical experts to discuss the data, which he felt indicated that doctors were prescribing more and more opioids without adequately monitoring patients. This was probably true: Claire Trescott, MD, in charge of overseeing primary care at Group Health in Seattle, has observed that treating pain patients is time-consuming and difficult because of common complicating factors such as depression and anxiety—and is not necessarily adequately compensated by insurers. Therefore, instead of focusing on the underlying condition causing the pain, doctors would often "end up chasing pain," she told *The New York Times*.

Official Recommendation

DR. FRANKLIN'S FINDINGS led in 2007 to an official state recommendation that doctors refer patients on high doses of pain medicine for further evaluation if their underlying condition was not improving. The recommendation set a specific level—the equivalent of one hundred twenty milligrams of morphine a day—above which patients were to be referred.

Doctors widely ignored the recommendation as long as it remained advisory. But in 2011, the state legislature made it a law—and suddenly the controversies about pain treatment were front-and-center. No one claimed there was any good reason for the arbitrary one hundred twenty mg limitation on pain medicine; even some supporters of the law said there was little evidence for the number. But they argued that it was necessary to start somewhere. Charles Chabal, MD, was quoted in the *Times* as calling the law "a necessary evil."

"Necessary" is debatable; "evil" is not, at least to pain patients. With one stroke, the state legislature forced uncounted numbers of chronic-pain sufferers into limbo, essentially telling them to reduce their use of quality-of-life-preserving medicines or jump through hoops—figuratively; they could scarcely do so literally—to get medication to make their everyday lives and activities bearable.

No one claimed there was any good reason for the arbitrary 120 mg limitation on pain medicine.

There is legitimate medical concern about the widespread use of opioids for chronic pain. Until the mid-1990s, the drugs were used mostly in end-of-life care or for postoperative or cancer treatment. But as pain experts became more familiar with the medicines' effectiveness—and pharmaceutical companies stepped up their advocacy of the drugs—the use of opioids grew dramatically. The medications understandably became an important weapon in doctors' treatment arsenal, argued Russell K. Portenoy, MD, chairman of pain medicine and palliative care at Beth Israel Medical Center in New York City: "I don't think opioids need to be thought of any differently than any other therapies." But other pain experts disagreed, with Jane C. Ballantyne, MD, in Seattle, saying the "mission to help people in pain" had been compromised because "the long-term outcomes for many of these patients are appalling, and it is ending up destroying their lives."

Making Life Bearable

WHO SAYS SO? Not the patients, who insist that far from destroying their lives, the drugs are the only thing making them bearable. But patients may not be fully aware of the very real consequences of long-term use of narcotic painkillers, especially in high doses: sleep apnea, increased falls and hip fractures in the elderly, and, in extreme cases, fatal overdoses. In less-extreme cases, there is sharply reduced production of hormones, including sex hormones, and there can be an overall decline in physical and mental functionality: C. Richard Chapman, MD, director of the Pain Research Center at the University of Utah, told the *Times* that "it is not just our sex lives that go away; it is our ability to get things done."

Indeed, the Centers for Disease Control and Prevention, which—unlike many other government agencies involved in the drug-overdose issue—does employ top-quality doctors, has urged doctors to use opioids with greater care. And Dr. Ballantyne says problems with the Washington state law are "teething pains," which will resolve in time or be fixed by the politicians. This, however, is small comfort to the people whose everyday activities are severely compromised by something far more serious and debilitating than teething pain.

The Centers for Disease Control and Prevention has urged doctors to use opioids with greater care.

But Dr. Ballantyne does have a point about the negative effects of high-dose, long-term opioid use, quite apart from the possibility of abuse of the medications. Logically, the best alternative to cracking down on prescription drug abuse without interfering with patients' genuine need for the medicines would seem to be focusing on patients who might abuse the medications and weeding them out or paying much closer attention to them. But this is difficult, time-consuming and costly, and while it has been tried only sporadically over the past two decades, there is no strong evidence that it has worked. And there *is* evidence that at least some patients with severe chronic pain can get along with lower doses of opioids than they have been given in recent years—or can do without them altogether if adequate alternative treatment is provided.

Group Health, which treats more than four hundred thousand patients at two dozen clinics in Washington state, has taken to carefully overseeing how doctors prescribe drugs. One Group Health patient who was using high-dose opioids plus methadone found that, after her Group Health doctor shepherded her through a significant reduction in her pain medicines, she became more sociable, talkative and relaxed, and more mentally alert, despite her pain. Group Health says it cut the percentage of patients on high-dose opioids in half in a four-year period, and reduced the average daily dose by one-third among patients who regularly use the medicines.

But as Roger Chou, MD, associate professor of medicine and medical informatics & clinical epidemiology at Oregon Health and Science University in Portland, pointed out, "You can't just take things away. You have to give patients alternatives." And this is precisely where the heavy-handed government crackdown on pain medicines—and the medically uninformed actions of politicians in Washington state and elsewhere—fall short. The patients are absent from the equation, or are at best an afterthought. Patients taken off opioids

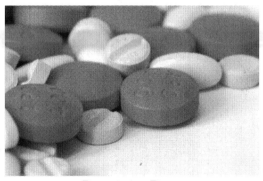

Prescription Drugs

will experience severe withdrawal symptoms and may need addiction-treatment drugs for many years—who supervises them, and who pays for their medicines?

Danish researchers published a study saying that chronic-pain patients getting nondrug treatments recover four times as quickly as those on opioids, and that is a very positive finding—but who creates those alternative treatments, implements them, manages them and, again, pays for them? Emphasizing nondrug approaches such as

You can't just take things away. You have to give patients alternatives.
—Roger Chou, M.D.

physical therapy and counseling, which is what Dr. Ballantyne advocates, may make sense in a controlled environment and for some patients, but is no more a panacea than are opioids. And who decides which patients get which treatment, who sees them and talks with them regularly, who determines when pain is just too severe *as experienced by the patient* to be handled without drugs? Within a largely self-contained system such as Group Health, it may be possible to monitor patients closely and have them seen regularly and repeatedly by doctors aware of their needs and physical conditions, and concerned with balancing opioid use against quality-of-life issues—but what of the vast majority of patients who are not in groups of this sort?

It is hard to argue with Dr. Ballantyne's assertion that there are better alternatives than high-dose opioids for many patients. But it is also hard to argue with Dr. Portenoy, who says that while there are certainly risks associated with opioid use, that is no excuse for an arbitrary dosage threshold imposed on doctors by politically motivated Washington state legislators—or for a state law that conspicuously does *not* contain a system designed to evaluate the impact of the law on patient health and care.

Florida's Situation

ALL THE WAY ACROSS THE UNITED STATES, what happens to chronic-pain sufferers in Florida, which does not have a law like the one in Washington state and which was certainly a mecca for pill mills and drug abuse until law enforcement started to crack down? In mid-2012, Florida Department of Law Enforcement spokesman Keith Kameg proudly said the state strike force had closed two hundred fifty-four pill mills and arrested about three thousand people, including forty-six doctors. There is, unsurprisingly, widespread support in Florida for restrictions on opioids in the name of reducing crime—just as there is inevitably widespread support among voters for raising taxes on people other than themselves.

The patients who *need* the opioids have done some organizing of their own, for example through the nonprofit advocacy group Fight for Pain Care Action Network in Lithia, Florida. But patients with an ongoing need for pain-controlling medication will always *Patients with chronic pain and an ongoing need for pain-controlling medication will always be a minority.* be a minority, and this gives the government essentially a free hand to crack down in a way that turns desperate people into mere "collateral damage." Paul Sloan, who owns two licensed pain-management clinics in Florida, says the DEA is intimidating people at every step of the medication supply chain: "There isn't a doctor, a pharmacist or a wholesaler in Florida that is not terrified of the Drug Enforcement Administration." And that, of course, is exactly what the DEA wants: a "chilling effect" that will lead to more self-policing and also make it clear that the federal government will not tolerate prescription drug abuse. What is left out of the equation, though, is the human cost of the crackdown. Sloan says, "I am just beside myself dealing with patients who can't get their medications."

Is there a happy medium? Is there a way to stop prescription drug abuse while allowing legitimate patients to get the medicines they need, and legitimate clinics and pharmacists to dispense them? The answer, in theory, is yes; in practice, though, the answer is no—since there is no government agency charged with finding such a balance.

9

Abuse Beyond Opioids

Opioids get most of the attention in discussions of prescription drug abuse, because of their potency and the extent to which they are prescribed—and because government crackdowns are highly publicized. But they are scarcely the only legitimate medications that are misused inadvertently by people consuming overdoses or by abusers trying to obtain the drugs' effects for pleasure. In fact, *non*prescription drugs can be subject to abuse, just as prescribed ones can. A good example is the nonprescription decongestant pseudoephedrine; its abuse potential explains the heavy-handed government attack on it, detailed in Chapter 3. Despite the fact that the government used a sledgehammer rather than a more-delicate tool on pseudoephedrine, it is important to realize that the medicine does have real abuse potential. The diversion of this substance into criminal activity for the manufacture of methamphetamine is well known—and it can also be abused by people who take it for nonmedical reasons.

Pseudoephedrine's Effects

PSEUDOSPHEDRINE CAUSES rapid heart rate, increased blood pressure and an excited, hyperactive feeling. Some people like those effects and take pseudoephedrine to obtain them. Others may use the substance in an attempt to lose weight, because its effects are similar to those of *ephedra*, also known as *ma huang*, a naturally occurring substance used in Chinese medicine. Ephedra was a popular weight-loss drug until it was banned in the United States near the start of the 21st century after being linked to some sixteen thousand adverse events, including heart attacks, strokes, seizures, and numerous deaths. Ephedra is chemically similar to amphetamines and can suppress the appetite and increase metabolism. Pseudoephedrine is close enough to ephedra in its effects so that some people use it in the absence of a way to obtain ephedra itself.

Ephedra is chemically similar to amphetamines and can suppress appetite and increase metabolism.

Furthermore, some athletes have been reported to abuse pseudoephedrine to help them get excited and pumped up before a competition. There have been cases of people taking significantly more than the recommended dose to try to increase the hyperactivity and excitability that pseudoephedrine can produce—but this is highly dangerous. It can lead to heart palpitations, irregular heart rhythms known as arrhythmias, and even to heart attacks.

Any medicine is subject to abuse, and you may have abused medications yourself—under the government definition of abuse—without even being aware of it. Suppose, for example, you are prescribed a pain medicine after minor surgery and given enough for a week—but you feel well enough to stop taking it after three days. Suppose you keep whatever you have left—and then, some time later, you

Any medicine is subject to abuse.

fall and hurt yourself. Aspirin or acetaminophen does
not relieve your pain—and then you remember that
you have some of the prescription medicine left. So you
use it. *You have just become a prescription drug abuser* by
taking medicine for a condition for which it was not
prescribed. Never mind that it was prescribed for you in
the first place—it was not prescribed at the specific time
you took it, for the specific condition for which you
used it. That, officially, is prescription drug abuse.

Benzodiazepine Abuse

THIS SORT OF ABUSE—or "misuse," a less pejorative
term—is not what federal officials normally mean when
they talk about the problem of improper use of medications, but it is worth realizing that by official government standards, pretty much everyone is or has been
a medication abuser. And in that context, the abuse
of benzodiazepines—sedatives such as diazepam, best
known as Valium®, and chlordiazepoxide, best known
as Librium®—is particularly common. Abusive use of
benzodiazepines produces effects similar to those of
intoxication caused by drinking too much alcohol—effects known to be attractive to many people, given the
numbers who over-imbibe occasionally or regularly.
These medicines may be taken as pills or ingested
through the nose—or even intravenously, by injection,
although this is less common. Benzodiazepines tend to
be abused in addition to other drugs—that is, people
who abuse other drugs often add benzodiazepines to the
other ones they take. For example, one study in India
found that fifty percent to sixty percent of heroin addicts also used benzodiazepines.

Benzodiazepines are a rather large class of drugs, and their abuse potential varies. The faster the plasma level of the drug rises after it is taken, the greater the intoxicating effect, and therefore the more likely the drug

Speed of onset is not the only criterion for misuse.

will be abused—benzodiazepines that take effect quickly are abused more often. The members of this class with the fastest onset of effect are alprazolam, sold as Xanax® and under other brand names; diazepam, best known as Valium®; flunitrazepam, sold as Rohypnol® and under other names; flurazepam, sold as Dalmadorm® or Dalmane®; lorazepam, sold as Ativan® and under other names; and temazepam, sold as Restoril® and under other names. Two other fast-onset benzodiazepines are less frequently abused, because they remain active for only an hour or less, which defeats much of the purpose of using them for nonmedical reasons. They are midazolam, known as Dormicum® and under other names, and triazolam, sold as Halcion® or Rilamir®.

Speed of onset is not, however, the only criterion for misuse. The four most commonly misused benzodiazepines in the United States are alprazolam, clonazepam, lorazepam and diazepam. The second of those, clonazepam—sold as Klonopin® and under other names—has only intermediate speed of onset; but it remains active in the body for up to twelve hours, longer than any other benzodiazepine.

Significant Dangers

THE DANGERS OF benzodiazepine misuse should not be underestimated. Between thirty percent and fifty percent of alcoholics are also thought to be abusers of benzodiazepines. Benzodiazepine abuse increases risk-taking behaviors, including unprotected sex and the sharing of needles among abusers who take benzodiazepines intravenously. Abuse is associated with blackouts, memory loss, aggression, violence, criminal activity, and a form of chaotic behavior related to paranoia. Benzodiazepines, like barbiturates and alcohol, create severe physical dependence with long-term use, which can lead to serious physical and mental withdrawal consequences. The list of withdrawal symptoms is a long one:

Benzodiazepine Withdrawal Symptoms

Depression	Objects seems to move
Shaking	Feeling faint
Appetite loss	Noise sensitivity
Muscle twitching	Peculiar taste
Memory loss	Pins and needles
Motor impairment	Touch sensitivity
Nausea	Sore eyes
Muscle pains	Hallucinations
Dizziness	Smell sensitivity

Furthermore, because benzodiazepines are often used in combination with alcohol, barbiturates, opioids or tricyclic antidepressants, their misuse can lead to coma, respiratory depression and death. They are also highly dangerous when used with sedating antipsychotics, anticonvulsants or antihistamines. Fatal overdoses from benzodiazepines alone are not common, but in certain groups, especially the elderly and people with chronic illnesses, they do occur.

Like opioids, benzodiazepines are very frequently prescribed drugs. This means there is a large supply of them accessible both to people who need them and to those seeking them in order to misuse them. However, the government treats them differently from opioids from a legal standpoint, and this is one major reason that more at-
*B*ecause benzodiazepines are often used in combination with other substances, their misuse can lead to coma, respiratory depression and death. tention is paid to opioid misuse than to benzodiazepine misuse. The Drug Enforcement Administration maintains a list of five classes of "controlled substances," ranging from Schedule I (the most tightly controlled) to Schedule V (least tightly). Schedule I is supposed to include only high-potential-abuse drugs without any valid medical use, although this schedule is also used for purely political rather than health-related purposes—marijuana, for example, is a Schedule I drug even though it has demonstrated medical efficacy and is legal for medical purposes under the laws of many states and, ironically, Washington, D.C.

The Drug Schedules

OPIOIDS ARE Schedule II drugs, which puts them in the same class as methadone, morphine, amphetamines and cocaine—which escapes Schedule I because it is used as a topical anesthetic. The Schedule II classification is not medically determined—the drugs have widely varying natures and uses. Interestingly, though, benzodiazepines are Schedule IV drugs, which the government says means that they have low abuse potential and that abuse may lead only to *limited* physical or

psychological dependence. Among drugs on Schedule
IV along with benzodiazepines are the insomnia treatment zolpidem, known as Ambien®; the sleep apnea
and narcolepsy treatment modafinil, sold as Provigil®;
and certain antidiarrheals.

From a medical standpoint, these drug classifications
sometimes make sense and sometimes do not; there is
no overall medical rationale governing them, and they
are as much instruments of social policy and political philosophy as of medicine. But they certainly have
medical *consequences*. For example, one longstanding
debate about combination opioids, such as Vicodin®,
Lortab® and Norco®, involves whether to classify them
as Schedule II or Schedule III. Under a Schedule II list-
ing, the drugs could not be prescribed for six months at
a time—only for three. And doctors prescribing them
could not call in or fax a prescription—patients would
have to bring a written prescription to the pharmacy.

For people in chronic pain, this is no small matter. The very people who cannot function in daily life
without the aid of these medicines would, under Schedule II, have to get to their doctors twice as frequently to
pick up written prescriptions, and make twice as many
trips to the pharmacy—two potentially significant
hardships for people in chronic, severe pain. There is
also a stigma associ-
ated with Schedule II
that is not attached to
Schedule III—not only
for patients but also for

*From a medical standpoint,
these drug classifications
sometimes make sense and
sometimes do not.*

doctors. Doctors would likely become more reluctant
to prescribe drugs that are moved from Schedule III to
Schedule II.

That is exactly the point, according to proponents of using the drug schedules to fight prescription drug abuse. Doctors *should* hesitate to prescribe these medicines, especially for longer-term use, and should move patients to other medications that are less likely to be abused, if not by the patients then by others. This is the sort of ongoing tug-of-war that prescription drug abuse creates in the medical and political spheres. And again and again, the people who really need these medicines are caught in the middle.

Any drug can potentially be abused, and the consequences can be severe and even dire—fatalities have been reported from overdoses of Tylenol® 3, which combines acetaminophen with a modest 30 milligrams of codeine. A reasonable and rational consideration of prescription drug abuse requires looking not at the drugs as enablers of abuse but at the factors that cause a small percentage of people to misuse the medications, resulting in significant and sometimes extreme restrictions on the medicines' use by people who genuinely need them. Reason and rationality, however, can be hard to come by in a situation seen as a political hot button and a moral imperative, as if a "war" on drugs is ever winnable. Logic says such victory is impossible—as long as the drugs exist, some people will abuse them. But logic does not necessarily govern societal attitudes or government policies.

10

Abuse Sneaks In

Most people find it hard to think of themselves as prescription drug abusers under the government's definition—but as we have seen, it is very easy to fall within the boundaries that the government sets, even if all you do is take some of your own leftover medication at some time after it has been prescribed, for some condition for which it was not originally intended. No one is likely to come knocking at your door and threatening to arrest you for this sort of drug misuse, but thinking about the narrowness of the definition of "prescription drug abuse" that the government uses can help you understand the level of frustration experienced by people who genuinely need medications, but cannot get them because the government defines them as "abusers" rather than as patients whose severe chronic pain requires potent medicines to make life manageable.

Even if the government overreaches in the name of its "war" on drug abuse, the fact is that abuse is a real issue and a real problem.

The government overreaches in the name of its "war" on drug abuse. But the fact is that abuse is a real issue and a real problem. And it *is* possible to become an abuser of prescription drugs without wanting or intending to. Knowing whether you or someone you care about is predisposed to abuse prescription drugs, or may even be abusing them already—without necessarily intending to—is important. This knowledge makes it possible to see a doctor or seek other medical help or counseling, if necessary, to prevent a downward spiral. The following *may* be signs that you or someone you care about could be or could become a prescription drug abuser.

General Signs of Abuse

Taking more of a medicine than the doctor prescribed—for instance, a pain pill every two hours instead of every four.

Consistently using up the prescribed medicine and needing to ask for more.

Losing prescriptions frequently, so more must be written.

Seeking prescriptions for the same drug from more than one doctor.

Depending on which medicine is involved, feeling or appearing to be "high," unusually energetic, or sedated.

Excessive mood swings—beyond what you or the other person has experienced in the past—or hostility.

Poor decision making or difficulty making decisions at all—again, if this is beyond what has previously been typical.

Overuse of any prescription drug may lead to these symptoms, but there are also symptoms unique to specific classes of drugs. If you suspect someone you care about is misusing medication, but are not sure what type of medicine is involved, look for additional symptoms caused by particular drugs.

Opioid Abuse Symptoms

Constipation

Depression

Low blood pressure

Decreased breathing rate

Confusion

Sweating

Poor coordination

Sedative and Anti-Anxiety Medicine
Abuse Symptoms

Drowsiness

Confusion

Unsteady walking

Poor judgment

Involuntary, rapid eye movements

Dizziness

Symptoms of Stimulant Abuse

Weight loss

Agitation

Irritability

Insomnia

High blood pressure

Irregular heartbeat

Restlessness

Impulsive behavior

We all may experience some of these symptoms from time to time. Interpreting the symptoms depends on the "baseline" of each individual. If you or the person about whom you are concerned is normally restless, there must be a significant increase in restlessness for this to have meaning; if you or the person you care about is usually somewhat clumsy, the level of poor coordination must be significantly greater than is typical for it to be potentially meaningful.

A Judgment Call

EVALUATING POSSIBLE SYMPTOMS is always going to be a judgment call. It is worth noting that some of these so-called "abuse indicators" are actually in line with *normal* uses of prescription medications. For example, deodorized tincture of opium, known as DTO, is legitimately used for control of severe diarrhea, and is so potent that it can easily cause constipation. So if someone with a prescription for DTO develops constipation, that may just mean that the medicine is working properly—not that it is being abused. The nuances matter—

and are precisely what the government makes no effort to identify or apply in its handling of prescription drug abuse or drugs in general. When evaluating yourself or someone who matters to you, though, nuance is crucial.

As hard as it can be to decide that you or someone you care about is or may be abusing prescription drugs, it can be even more difficult to find medical advice or treatment. The social stigma

Some "abuse indicators" are actually in line with normal uses of prescription medications.

associated with drug abuse can make it embarrassing to admit that you or someone important to you needs help. The idea of talking to a doctor about this may seem humiliating, resulting in failure to seek help early enough for the condition to be treated effectively. But early handling of prescription drug abuse is important— catching it before it turns into full-blown addiction makes treatment much easier and significantly reduces the risk of serious problems.

It may help to repeat to yourself, as often as necessary, that medical professionals are trained to help, not judge. And it can also help to realize that prescription drug abuse happens for a variety of reasons, not just because people want to "get high," experiment with the mental effects of a medicine, or be accepted by a peer group.

Reasons Abuse Occurs

To relax

Relieving tension

Appetite suppression

Improving concentration

Boosting alertness

Seeking to improve performance

Self-evaluation on these factors, as difficult as it may be, can be very helpful in providing reassurance to yourself or someone else that there is not necessarily a "moral failing" or "succumbing to peer pressure" underlying prescription drug abuse.

One way or another, it is important to get help for prescription drug abuse as soon as it is identified. The consequences of waiting until things go further downhill can be severe. Opioids can cause low blood pressure, a slowed breathing rate—even to the point that breathing can stop altogether—and coma. Sedatives can cause memory problems, low blood pressure, and—in overdose cases—coma or death; but stopping them quickly, even if you can do it, can cause serious withdrawal symptoms, such as seizures. And stimulants can raise body temperature to dangerous levels as well as cause heart problems, seizures, tremors, hallucinations, aggression and paranoia. All these drugs are potent and can be truly dangerous.

One way or another, it is important to get help for prescription drug abuse as soon as it is identified.

Once you convince yourself or the person you care about to see a doctor to discuss prescription drug abuse, prepare a list of your concerns and symptoms and put some questions down on paper so you remember to ask them.

Questions for Your Doctor

What are my treatment options?

How long will treatment take?

Would it be better to have a specialist handle my treatment?

How will other health conditions be managed during treatment?

Elements of Treatment

THE FORM OF TREATMENT varies depending on which drugs are being misused or abused, but talk therapy is almost always a key element. This may be individual, group or family counseling, depending on circumstances—but some sort of therapeutic talk is almost always recommended. Medications may be used as well to help in withdrawal from opioids or sedatives, but not from stimulants—there are no approved drugs for stimulant withdrawal.

Medicines used in opioid cases include *buprenorphine, Suboxone®*—which is buprenorphine plus *naloxone*—and/or *methadone*, and sometimes *clonidine*, a blood-pressure drug that can help ease withdrawal symptoms. Mood stabilizers and anti-anxiety medications of various types are typically used during withdrawal from sedative abuse, because it can take weeks or months to go through withdrawal as the sedative doses are gradually tapered and then stopped.

As for stimulants, tapering is used there, too, but in the absence of medicines that specifically help ease withdrawal symptoms, doctors usually treat whatever symptoms occur in individual cases—such as sleep disturbance, appetite problems and mood issues.

More important than the medicines used in treating prescription drug abuse is something that doctors can sometimes provide but cannot prescribe—*understanding*. There is a constant undercurrent of the judgmental, of harshness, about government approaches to prescription drug abuse, but the law-enforcement model—while it makes sense

The law-enforcement model is wholly out of place in a family or personal setting.

for criminal activity—is wholly out of place in a family or personal setting. Some people do better by reaching out to family members and close friends, asking for help and support in a difficult time. Others prefer to lean on employee-assistance programs at work…churches or religious organizations…support groups, either in person or online…or 12-step programs, such as Narcotics Anonymous.

These sources of help are very different and operate in very different ways, but what they all have in common is nonjudgmental emotional and psychological backing for people struggling with a difficult personal situation that can best be handled with understanding rather than in a government-style punitive way. If, for example, someone you love shows signs of prescription drug abuse, it is far better for you to approach him or her with compassion and patience, showing that you care about his or her well-being, than to "come on strong" and demand that the person clean up his or her act and get some sort of help. The in-tense approach will only bring on denial and anger—which indeed may result from *any* attempt to *Some people do better by reaching out to family members and close friends, asking for help and support in a difficult time.*

bring up the subject, but which are far more likely to emerge if the discussion is handled harshly.

Winning the Fight

PRESCRIPTION DRUG ABUSE can be fought success-fully at the individual and family level, even if it is like-ly always to remain a societal problem. There are seven simple steps that you can take to prevent prescription drug abuse by someone you care for—or by yourself.

Preventing Prescription Drug Abuse

1. *Be sure the doctor prescribes the right medi-cation.* Make sure your doctor fully understands your condition and symptoms. Provide a list of all your current prescriptions—plus over-the-counter medicines, herbs and supplements, and informa-tion on any alcohol and drug use. Ask directly whether a medicine that he or she may pre-scribe is potentially addictive and whether, if so, there are ways to make abuse and addiction less likely—for example, by prescribing an extended-release version.

2. *Talk to your doctor regularly* to be sure the medicine you are using is working properly and that you are taking the right dose.

3. *Follow directions for use carefully.* Do not change dosage on your own, and do not stop taking the medicine or double up on it if you miss a dose unless your doctor says it is all right to do that. In particular, if a pain medicine does not seem to be helping your pain, tell your doctor— do not simply take more.

4. *Know the effects and side effects of every medicine you are prescribed,* so you understand what to expect and do not overreact to perceived problems.

5. *Never use another person's prescription.* People are different—even if your condition is similar to the other person's, his or her medicine may be wrong for you, or may be the right medicine but at the wrong dosage.

6. *Use your own medicines only for the purposes for which they are intended.* Safely dispose of any that may be left after an illness has run its course or after pain, such as post-surgical pain, has disappeared. Saving leftover medicine "just in case" makes it all too easy to take the medication in the future for an inappropriate purpose.

7. *If you have chronic pain requiring ongoing use of opioids*—or any chronic condition because of which you need to take medicine on an ongoing basis—do not hesitate to speak up. Tell your doctor how you feel; explain if the medicine is not working at a certain dosage (but do not increase

it yourself); talk to a knowledgeable pharmacist about alternative medications or ones that may work in combination with what you are already taking; and explore alternatives for chronic pain, from the naturopathic, herbal and chiropractic to acupuncture and other Oriental approaches, from dietary alteration to medical use of marijuana.

There is no shame in having chronic pain. There is no shame in needing medication for a long time, even for life, so that you can live more comfortably and be happier and more productive. Prescription drug abuse is real, is damaging, and is a significant societal problem. But the ongoing use of potent medicines by people who really need them is *not* the problem. Indeed, heavy-handed government sweeps that catch patients and well-meaning pharmacists in nets designed for criminals are more dangerous than the drug "abuse" the sweeps are designed to control.

You have rights, including the right to live as comfortable and pain-free a life as possible. Remember that, and insist that your healthcare practitioners—and, if need be, law-enforcement personnel—understand and respect those rights. Take control of your body and take control of your life, and insist that those with whom you interact treat you and your needs with respect. Do not ignore the realities that make prescription drug abuse a costly drain on society, but do not get swept up in hysteria or a punishment orientation that prevents

There is no shame in needing medication for a long time, even for life, so that you can live more comfortably and be happier and more productive.

people who really need strong medicine from receiving the treatment that helps them function. The pain you relieve may be your own—if not right now, then at some point in the future.

11

How Abuse Happens

It is easy to think of prescription drug abuse as something that happens to "them," to other people who are weak or have some sort of physical, mental or even moral flaw that makes them prone to dependency and addiction. This sort of thinking, though, is facile and unfair, and does nothing to explain how prescription drug abuse has become such a significant societal problem. If it were merely a matter of a very few individuals misusing prescription drugs, it would be much easier to manage. While it is true that a small *percentage* of people taking prescription drugs will become abusers, that is still a large *number* of people, because there are so many drugs that can be abused and they are prescribed so widely. For example, more than fifteen million Americans admit using a prescription drug for non-medical reasons at least once during the previous year.

The fact is that these drugs are *prescription* medicines for a reason: they are very powerful, highly addictive, and have significant systemic ef-

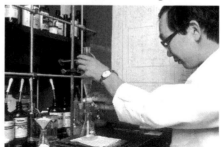

Drug synthesis in a laboratory

fects. Abuse can happen in several ways. Sometimes
people seek out a drug's effects or side effects rather
than its curative properties. But in many cases, it
is simply a matter of overusing a drug to get more
of the effect it is supposed to have. The easiest
instance of this to understand is pain relief. Potent
opioids are prescribed to help people cope with
severe pain. Doctors know that, to prevent physical dependency on the drugs—that is, addiction—the
medicines should be taken with a specific frequency
during the day and for only a set number of days.
But pain does not occur or disappear on a neat
schedule, and it is entirely understandable that if
pain recurs sooner than expected, or if a person's
individual pain tolerance is lower than average, it
will be tempting to take an extra dose of medicine,
or to take the next dose sooner than called for on
the label.

Abuse and Misuse

THIS IS A COMMON FORM OF DRUG ABUSE—and
the word "misuse" probably fits it better, since it
does not have the same negative connotations. Unfortunately, a combination of physical and psychological factors involved in this type of misuse can cause
it to continue over time, and can cause use of the
drug to increase to the point of addiction—that is,
of physical dependency enforced by withdrawal symptoms if a person tries to cut back. Misuse or abuse
may progress to addiction—or may not. But the risk
is there, and the behaviors associated with prescription drug abuse come in many forms and many
levels of severity.

Is My Loved One an Opioid Abuser?

Instructions: Thinking about your loved one, friend, or colleague, read each item carefully. Using a scale from 1 to 5—where 1 = "rarely" and 5 = "usually"—rate how often the statement describes your loved one or friend's behavior.

My friend or loved one:

___ 1. Uses up meds more quickly than the prescription says to use them.

___ 2. Goes to the doctor for a new script before using up the old one.

___ 3. Goes to multiple doctors for the same meds.

___ 4. Takes meds for something other than for what they were prescribed.

___ 5. Increases the dose if the prescribed amount is not helping.

___ 6. Takes someone else's meds.

___ 7. Loses or misplaces meds and has to get replacements.

___ 8. Has mood swings when taking meds.

___ 9. Talks frequently about meds.

___ 10. Uses meds to relieve tension and relax.

___ 11. Needs stronger pain relievers than what others use.

___ 12. Needs more meds than the doctor prescribes.

___ 13. Enjoys the effects of meds.

___ 14. Has trouble making decisions while taking meds.

___ 15. Looks forward to taking meds.

Score:

15: Your loved one uses prescription drugs responsibly.

16-30: While your loved one generally uses prescription drugs responsibly, he or she is a prescription drug abuser by the government's definition—although not in the opinion of most people.

31-45: Your loved one is in danger of becoming a prescription drug abuser. Encourage him or her to talk to the doctor about use of prescription drugs to get the maximum benefit from them with the lowest likelihood of harm or dependency.

46-60: Strong likelihood of abuse. He or she must discuss drug use with a doctor to find ways to prevent full-scale abuse and possible addiction.

61-75: Serious danger of becoming drug dependent. Guidance from a doctor is necessary as soon as possible—you may want to contact the doctor yourself if your loved one does not do so. This behavior is dangerous.

What the Score Means

PRESCRIPTION DRUGS SHOULD BE USED only at the time they are prescribed, for the specific condition for which they are prescribed—and should be properly discarded if you do not use them up. By government standards, even the slightest deviation from this equals abuse—which makes practically everyone at least a low-level abuser.

The real medical issue has to do with obtaining more drugs than you need, using them for purposes other than those for which they are prescribed, and enjoying the effects they have—as opposed to simply using them to get through an injury or illness more comfortably.

If in doubt about whether you may be abusing prescription drugs—or misusing them, a less pejorative term—talk to your doctor. This may be difficult—but remember that your doctor will not condemn you for your behavior. A doctor's job is to help, not to judge.

Real-World Dangers

THE QUIZ GIVES each question equal weight for scoring purposes, but it should be clear that in the real world, certain behaviors are more indicative of prescription drug abuse than others. Someone who steals medicines or sells them to other people is far more likely to be a prescription drug abuser than someone who simply holds onto prescribed drugs instead of discarding them, or uses pain medicine left over after a tooth extraction to cope with a severe headache—which is a form of taking medicine for a purpose other than the one for which it was prescribed.

It is important to understand that there are both physical and psychological benefits to using prescription drugs more often than recommended; otherwise, prescription drug abuse would not be an issue. Physically, the medicines relieve symptoms that would otherwise be at least inconvenient and at most incapacitating. Psychologically, they make users feel better able to cope with everyday life—more empowered,

more in control of themselves. It is the combination
of these factors that makes prescription drug abuse
so tempting and so insidious. Users experience effects that they perceive in a highly positive way—not
realizing just how severe the negative effects of the
drugs can be, and in fact not experiencing those
negatives at all for some time.

Effects of Addictive Prescription Drugs

OxyContin®: This time-release painkiller—chemical
    name *oxycodone*—produces intense euphoria when
    snorted or injected. Highly subject to overdose,
    it has a long list of side effects, from memory
    loss and nightmares to anxiety, heavy sweating,
    abdominal pain, diarrhea, shallow breathing, low
    blood pressure, even circulatory collapse and
    respiratory arrest—which can be fatal.

Demerol®: Inhibits the area of the brain that con-
    trols pain, producing feelings of euphoria. With-
    drawal can cause depression, fever, and suicidal
    thoughts.

Vicodin®: Produces strong euphoric feelings. Withdrawal
    leads to agitation, anxiety, insomnia, nausea and
    vomiting.

Percocet®: Contains oxycodone plus acetaminophen.
    A euphoria-producing drug, it can cause heart
    failure.

Darvocet®: Contains propoxyphene plus acetamino-
    phen. Used medically for somewhat less-serious
    pain than Percocet®, but can still bring euphoric
    feelings and cause withdrawal symptoms. The acet-
    aminophen in Percocet® and Darvocet® can cause
    liver disorders in people who overuse the drugs.

Ritalin®: A stimulant used for treatment of Attention Deficit/Hyperactivity Disorder, it is abused by people seeking to increase alertness and energy, and sometimes because one of its side effects is weight loss. Some people use it as a substitute for cocaine. It can cause significant changes in blood pressure and lead to psychotic episodes.

This is a very small sampling of commonly abused drugs—as we have seen, *any* drug can be abused, although not necessarily for these particular reasons. Addiction, the actual physical dependence on a drug, can start innocently, through use of a drug when you feel you really need it—rather than on the schedule for which your doctor prescribes it. Your doctor is surely aware of the dangers of these medicines, but still considers them the best way to treat you for a given condition at a given time.

Following the doctor's instructions is, in essence, managing the drugs' dangers. Still, it is very easy, for both physical and psychological reasons, to bend those instructions just a bit. For example, your doctor might prescribe a pain medicine to be taken every six to eight hours. But if your pain is so severe that you can barely stand it after four hours, you may take the next dose then—it is, after all, only a little early. Then you may take the medication yet again in four hours rather than six to eight. This is a common misuse or abuse pattern. It is understandable, but is an early sign that you are sliding into behavior that could eventually become addiction—being controlled by the drug.

From Doctor to Doctor

OF COURSE, taking the drug too often means you
will run out of it sooner than expected. This leads
people to ask doctors for additional prescriptions or
to go to a different doctor for the same medicine.
Many doctors, concerned about pain, will in fact
provide a renewal prescription, at least once, so that
you don't have to make an office visit. But they are
unlikely to keep doing so: they should insist you
return for a re-examination, at which time your doctor may change your pain medicine to a new one
or reduce the dose to be sure you do not become
dependent upon it.

Remember, *pain is not an objective symptom.* Doctors
routinely measure and test for many things, but the
degree to which you experience pain—your personal
pain tolerance—is not one of them. Considerable
progress has been made in at-
tempts to measure pain objec-
tively with functional magnetic
resonance imaging, but even
when reliable techniques to measure the *level* of pain are devel-
oped, they will be unable to determine the *perception*
of pain by each individual. People denied additional
medicines by one doctor may understandably seek
them from another if the pain seems severe or unbearable.

*Pain is not
    an objective
    symptom.*

To complicate matters further, patients who run
out of medicine when their doctor is away or un-
available may choose to or need to see a different
doctor, who may not know them and may not fully
comprehend their medical history—and may there-

fore be more willing to prescribe medication. This can set the stage for "doctor shopping." It all starts with pain, not with any moral failing. So identifying non-drug ways to cope with pain, especially as acute pain—from an injury or surgery, for example—diminishes over time, can be a valuable part of avoiding prescription drug abuse. The key is figuring out what non-drug methods work for you, and finding ways to use them even while continuing to take medication as your doctor recommends.

12

Helping Without Guilt

Because pain medicines, especially the powerful opioids, do their job so well, they make people feel better—that *is* their job. And who doesn't want to feel better? So it can be perfectly natural for someone to want to continue feeling well—and if taking a drug leads to that feeling, that is a powerful incentive to take it. This is one of those "slippery slope" issues, in which you start doing something that seems reasonable and soon find it becoming a bigger problem than the one you set out to solve.

Nor is it just opioids that result in drug-abusing behavior. Sometimes medicines prescribed to *counter* the side effects of opioids can themselves become problematical. For example, some people taking *Vicodin®* for pain experience nausea, and doctors sometimes prescribe *promethazine*—sold under such brand names as Phenergan® and *Prothiazine®*—to deal with the queasiness. Promethazine has a calming effect, not only relieving nausea but also producing an overall feeling of relaxation. So some patients develop a dependency, not on the opioid pain reliever, but on the anti-nausea

There is no single pattern of behavior that results in prescription drug abuse.

medicine designed to counteract the opioid's side effect. As with any prescription drug abuse, these people feel good while taking the drug and bad if they do not take it—leading to increased dependency. Upon attempted withdrawal, there are separate side effects, which in the case of promethazine can include anxiety, appetite loss, chills, nausea, diarrhea, increased heart rate, backache, and muscle and joint pains. It is a vicious cycle and a deeply dangerous one: pain leads to taking an opioid that produces nausea; the medicine to counteract the nausea, when overused, can lead to side effects including both pain and nausea.

It Isn't Easy

THE FACT IS that there is no single pattern of behavior that results in prescription drug abuse or even addiction to these medicines. If there were, there could be a prescription, so to speak, to deal with it. The reason that government at all levels flails about in its attempts to handle the problem is rooted in the individuality of circumstances that lead to the abuse.

And it is not just government that has trouble figuring out how to handle the issue—so do families. It tends to be the celebrity drug abusers who get most of the attention—the Michael Jacksons and Rush Limbaughs—but the greater tragedy is not that wealthy, much-indulged people become abusers, but that people who are simply trying to get through life from day to day can find themselves becoming victims of the very medicines that are intended to help them.

How Addiction Takes Hold

Addiction—the development of actual physical and mental dependence on drugs—is a result of a misperception of rewards and punishments. Behavior that produces positive feelings and effects gets reinforced and therefore increases; if it produces negative feelings and effects, it decreases. We experience this all the time in everyday life. We are social beings, and if we smile, others tend to smile back; that makes us feel good, so we smile more. That is positive reinforcement.

Addiction gains its power from negative reinforcement—actions that soothe or turn off a negative are rewarding. For example, having a headache is a negative. If you take aspirin

Behaviors that soothe pain or relieve anxiety tend to get repeated.

or acetaminophen and your headache goes away, you will probably reach for the same medicine the next time your head hurts. Any action that turns off something negative—a headache, in this example—provides negative reinforcement—a reward gained by removing a negative—and you are likely to repeat the same negative-relieving activity if you re-experience the same negative.

The danger is that each time you soothe or remove the negative, the pain-reducing action gets stronger and stronger, becoming a kind of super-habit or addiction that can take control of you.

When it comes to pain, it is important to be aware of the ways that you personally turn off negative emotions such as stress and worry.Because these methods are successful in soothing your worry, for example, they have power to control you. Understanding that psychological reality makes it easier to select more-beneficial, less-dangerous ways to fight all forms of pain. These may include deep breathing, relaxation techniques, listening to soothing music, positive self-talk, calling a friend, watching a funny movie or TV show to take advantage of the power of laughter, and so on. And discussing these options with your doctor can be helpful—then both of you will understand that your experience of pain is real and that you are making positive efforts to cope with it, not simply reaching unthinkingly for additional medication.

Signs of Abuse

A HISTORY OF DRUG ABUSE or addiction increases the chance that someone will abuse prescription drugs, but in the vast majority of cases, there is no such history. Abuse may not be an issue for you personally—but it may very well be one for a family member or close friend. In that case, there are things that you can watch for to determine whether someone you care about is abusing prescription medications.

Signs of Prescription Drug Abuse

Continued use of the drug after the condition for which it was prescribed is no longer present.

Complaining about vague symptoms to get additional prescriptions.

Having a lack of interest in treatment options other than medication.

Behavioral changes or mood swings beyond the
norm for that person—becoming depressed, agi-
tated, hostile, volatile, anxious, etc.

Developing a tolerance for a medicine, so more
is needed to get the desired effect, such as pain
relief.

Physical withdrawal symptoms if doses are
missed—often including flu-like symptoms, night
sweats, insomnia, and/or joint and muscle aches.

Withdrawing from social contact with friends,
family and acquaintances—especially those who
tell the person he or she has a problem.

Feeling Guilty

KNOWING JUST WHEN these behaviors indicate prescription drug abuse is difficult—especially so because
abuse is not an all-or-nothing phenomenon. The point
of the "Is My Loved One an Opioid Abuser?" quiz in
Chapter 11 is to show that a wide range of behaviors
can indicate prescription drug abuse. It is not as if a
medication user is always transformed suddenly into an
abuser—abuse can sneak up on you.

For example, it can be extremely difficult for friends
and family to realize that certain personality traits that
someone has always had have now become so accen-
tuated that they indicate that something is seriously
wrong. If someone has always been short-tempered,
how much *more* short-tempered must he or she become
for it to be a symptom of prescription drug abuse? There
is no easy answer. If someone tends to be anti-social,
at what point does his or her withdrawal become cause

for concern? There is no one-size-fits-all way to know; every person, every situation, is different.

Nevertheless, at some point the prescription drug abuser's behavior will reach a level that convinces family members and friends that something is seriously wrong. A common reaction at this point, if you are sure someone you care for is abusing prescription drugs, is to talk to the person about it—and what commonly happens then is that the person denies drug abuse and invokes a "blame game" that causes tremendous

Every person, every situation, is different.

feelings of guilt in anyone who would even suggest that he or she is an abuser. It is important to anticipate this reaction and understand where it comes from: if someone else is responsible for the abuser's behavior, then he or she does not have to take responsibility for it and find ways to change it.

Prescription drug abusers, once confronted with their behavior, can become aggressive in their own defense. They may argue that these are *prescribed* medicines they are using; their pain—or other condition for which the medication was given to them—is real and acknowledged by the doctor; they have a lower pain tolerance than other people; they have additional pressures in life that make them feel worse, so they need more than the prescribed amount of medicine; the person confronting them is a big part of the problem; in fact, they are not abusing prescription drugs at all, but are using them only as necessary to be able to function; how dare anyone try to understand how they feel and how much they need these medicines just to get through the day?

Buying into Guilt

THESE AND SIMILAR ARGUMENTS will often elicit guilt feelings and make it harder for you to be sure that abuse is really occurring. And the statements may contain a large enough grain of truth to derail your determination to confront the abuser. After all, the abuser *did* get the medicine by prescription and *does* have a real physical issue and *is* under a variety of pressures—and so on. If the net result is that you feel guilty bringing up the subject at all, the abuser gains more time with the drug—and will likely seek to gain even more by withdrawing from you because of your "unfounded suspicions."

What can you do at this stage? It is easy to say that you should not feel guilty—after all, you are in no way responsible for an abuser's decision to misuse prescription drugs. But you may still *feel* responsible. In fact, if you did not feel a close connection, you would not have confronted him or her in the first place. And a firm denial from the abuser may create self-doubt in you. Should you discuss your suspicions with other family members or friends, or with a doctor? But what if you are wrong? What if the person has withdrawn from you *because* you voiced unfounded suspicions—not because the withdrawal is itself a symptom of the abuse?

Difficult Decisions

DECIDING WHAT TO DO when you strongly suspect prescription drug abuse but cannot prove it is extremely difficult. It may be tempting to look the other way, letting the abuse escalate significantly before you are willing to say anything about it. The layer of guilt simply makes things more perplexing—if someone close to you is abusing prescription drugs, maybe you do have something to do with it. In fact, when you try to discuss the situation, the abuser may directly accuse *you* of being the reason he or she needs the drugs—just as alcoholics, confronted with *their* addiction, will often blame the people who warn them of the abyss into which they are falling.

There is no hard-and-fast rule that will let you say with certainty and finality that yes, someone you care about has become a prescription drug abuser. But at some point, no matter how much you want it *not* to be so, no matter how guilty you may feel for your own complicity—real or imagined—in the person's abuse, you will realize that something must be done.

Do's and Don'ts

Do not nag or preach—speak calmly and firmly.

Do not accept guilt for decisions the abuser is making.

Do not act as if prescription drug abuse is some sort of "disgrace"—it is not a moral failing.

Do not act holier-than-thou—you may not be prone to prescription drug abuse, but everyone has weaknesses of some sort.

Do not whine or say "if you loved me" to try to get the abuser to change behavior—abuse is a form of compulsion that cannot simply be controlled by will power.

Do learn about how abuse happens and what its effects are.

Do find out what role you may have in your loved one's prescription drug abuse—not to make yourself feel guilty, but to find positive changes that you yourself can make.

Do accept that you cannot "solve the problem" of your loved one's prescription drug abuse.

Do understand that if the abuser refuses to acknowledge the abuse, you *must* reach out to other people in order to help him or her.

Why Reach Out?

THE REASON FOR SOLICITING help from others to deal with your loved one's prescription drug abuse is that your loved one will likely resist anything you do on your own to try to change his or her behavior. Neither encouragement nor subtle threats will likely work. And if you escalate the threats, even to the point of saying you will cut off your relationship, you must follow through—because if you withdraw that threat, you undermine your own credibility and will feel helpless and, yes, guilty. Once it fully takes hold, prescription drug abuse, like the abuse of alcohol and illegal drugs, can be extremely difficult to fight. Fortunately, there is a technique you can use that has been employed with considerable success in dealing with alcohol and illegal-drug use. It can be one of the most helpful things you can do for someone you care about, and one of the most difficult: an intervention.

13

Love and Intervention

Drug abuse hurts relationships and undermines families. Prescription drug abuse, which may start after a loved one suffers a serious accident or illness and needs to be cared for and medicated for a considerable period of time, can be particularly devastating. The ill or injured person, needing strong medicine to cope with physical problems initially, may gradually become an abuser of the medication—so slowly that he or she may not even realize it, and others in the family may be equally unaware. By the time it starts to become clear that they have a problem, prescription drug abusers often blame family members, spouses, children, friends—anyone but themselves. And family members may well see themselves as enablers of the drug abuse—after all, they did care for the person during recovery and may even have made sure to obtain the prescribed medicines.

Blame and guilt can make you feel hopeless.

Show Love

IT IS ALL WELL AND GOOD to say that you should avoid blame and avoid blaming others—and not feel guilty about helping a loved one who has become a prescription drug abuser—but it is much easier to say that than to believe it. The thing about blame and guilt—and it *may* be helpful to realize this—is that they are counterproductive. They have no positive impact on the present or future. All they do is open the way to self-doubt, indecision, and inaction—they take attention away from what must be done to help the abuser.

Blame and guilt make you feel hopeless, make you believe there is nothing you can do to change the situation. They paralyze you. Feel guilty enough, feel sufficiently swamped by blame heaped on you by the abuser or by your own feelings, and you will lose hope and get stuck in take-no-action mode. That means your loved one will get no help and will not overcome the prescription-drug-abusing behavior, but will only get worse—and may descend into full-blown addiction and its extremely serious consequences.

Confronting prescription drug abusers often leads them to retreat further into isolation.

Two Attempts

COMPOUNDING THE DIFFICULTY is the fact that the two basic, opposite approaches that loved ones typically try with abusers are both equally likely to fail. Most people take a confrontational and accusatory approach, trying to intimidate an abuser and basically bully him or her into getting help. This is understandable, given the frustration you feel watching a loved one descend further into prescription drug abuse and maybe crossing the line into actual drug addiction. But this approach almost always backfires, driving the abuser into guilt-tripping you if possible and resenting you almost certainly—and pushing him or her further into isolation and communing with medications, not with you or other people.

Unfortunately, the opposite approach is no more likely to succeed. This involves being loving and caring, trying to convince abusers that they need help and that it is only because you care so much that you are telling them this—and that you really want to get them the help they need. Here the problem is that the abuser does not connect with what you say, does not see what the problem is or claims not to, and feels you are overreacting, "making a mountain out of a molehill," or simply not understanding his or her need for medication. The result is often the same as with the confrontational approach—the abuser retreats further into isolation from people like you who "just don't understand."

Getting Through

IT IS THEORETICALLY POSSIBLE to get through to prescription drug abusers who have not descended into full-blown addiction by talking to them in a way that gets them to break through their own denial. You may be able to question them—not lecture them—in a way that will lead them to conclude *on their own* that something has gone wrong and that they need help. Ideally, abusers questioned this way will go into treatment of their own volition. And if they do, the treatment is more likely to be successful than if they are forced into it.

However, finding the right way to get through to abusers so they go for help on their own is extremely difficult—even professionals have considerable trouble doing so. So you may very well *have* to force an abuser whom you care about into treatment. *It is useless to beat yourself up about needing to do this.* Try to hold that realization in your mind and heart—it will help you get beyond blame and guilt. Deciding to discard blame and guilt lets you tell a loved one, at the right time and in the right context, how concerned and worried you are—without assigning fault and without accepting it. You can take *responsibility* for matters in the past—perhaps for giving your loved one occasional extra doses of medicine to alleviate severe pain—but then you must move on to the future so you can help him or her move on as well.

Five Steps to Helping an Abuser

1. Figure out what drug he or she is abusing—or what combination of drugs. Knowing this will help you determine what can be done.

2. Learn each drug's positive effects, side effects, and the reasons abuse of it may be appealing. Knowing that one drug makes someone feel energized and another makes a person feel relaxed and at peace can help you figure out how to deal with the person's needs—making it easier for him or her to get through withdrawal.

3. Learn about abuse and addiction in general to understand what the person is and will be going through. This is especially important if you have never been an addict. It can help to think about possibly addictive behaviors of your own. How much coffee do you drink daily? Do you eat when you are not hungry? These can be addictive behaviors if you use them to cope with some sort of pain—such as work stress or family problems.

4. Find out the options for fighting your loved one's particular form of prescription drug abuse—which can range from medication changes to talk therapy to a formal detox program.

5. Get other friends and family members to help you—they may be just as concerned as you are, but not know what to say or do. Show those who are unaware of the situation why you are sure your loved one is abusing prescription drugs, and ask them to join you in approaching him or her. This is the foundation of an *intervention*, a drastic step that can be highly effective if properly managed.

Staging an Intervention

AN INTERVENTION is a *carefully planned* confrontation with a drug abuser, in which family, friends, appropriate colleagues, clergy members, doctors and others who care about the person confront him or her about the abuse and its consequences—and ask him or her to go into treatment immediately. The words *carefully planned* are crucial: this is not a spontaneous gathering in which well-meaning people try to convince a prescription drug abuser—who will likely be in denial and may very well become hostile—about the dangers of his or her behavior.

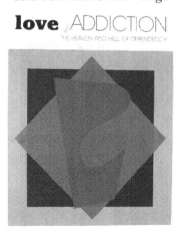

love ADDICTION
THE HEAVEN AND HELL OF DEPENDENCY

One key to a successful intervention is *specificity*. Since the prescription drug abuser will likely deny having a problem, the intervening people must provide specific examples of behaviors that show the person's addiction—and discuss the

A key to a successful intervention is specificity.

impact of those behaviors on the abuser and on family and friends. There must be specific plans for treatment as well—this is why it is so important to understand exactly what drugs are being abused and what their effects are. The abuser may very well agree to "go into treatment," but that is not enough—he or she must accept the specific treatment plan presented at the intervention, and must accept it *immediately*.

Why would abusers accept intervention-recommended treatment? Because there must be very serious consequences if they do not. Each friend and family member at the intervention must say specifically, and in as much detail as necessary, what he or she will do if the abuser refuses to accept the specific treatment around which the intervention is designed. And each person must be willing to follow through, whatever the emotional and other consequences may be, including feelings of guilt or of having betrayed the abuser. The abuser's parents, for example, might say they will stop visiting or stop providing financial support; a friend might say their regular nights out together will end; a colleague who regularly chooses the abuser as partner in complex projects might say this will no longer happen. These and other statements must not be made vindictively and must not be attributed to any sort of "moral flaw" in the abuser—all participants have to make it clear that it is *the behavior produced by the prescription drug abuse* that is leading them, regretfully and despite how much they care for the abuser, to make these difficult decisions.

It is crucial to be prepared to do what you say you will do. If, for example, a prescription drug abuser's wife says she will take the children and move into her parents' home with them if her husband does not enter a specified treatment program, she *must* do so—despite financial concerns and worries about what he might do to himself without her steadying hand. If she cannot be sure of following through, she should not name this consequence, because all she will do is undermine her own credibility and that of the others involved in the intervention.

When to Intervene

INTERVENTION IS MOST EFFCTIVE when the abuser does not yet understand the effects his or her behavior has on other people. The whole point of gathering multiple people in an intervention is to show the abuser just how wide-ranging and deep those effects are—and to provide moral support for the interveners themselves, since an intervention is emotionally trying and can be very difficult for all concerned.

Interventions are complicated as well as difficult, and it can be a good idea to consult a professional when planning one. Psychologists, medical doctors, mental-health counselors and some members of the clergy may be able to help plan an intervention or refer you to appropriate people—there are actually specialists known as *interventionists* who are experienced in the process. If

You must be prepared to do what you say you will do.

you believe there is any chance that your loved one will go beyond denial and verbal anger into violence or self-destructiveness because of the intervention, be sure to consult a professional and share your concerns.

Seven Steps of an Intervention

1. *Planning.* Form the group by speaking with family members, friends, the intervention professional, and others who will help, such as a doctor or counselor.

2. *Gather information.* All group members need to learn about the extent of the abuser's problem and find out about treatment options, then plan a specific treatment regimen.

3. *Form the team.* It may not be good for all group members to participate in the intervention—some may find it too difficult or may not be at their best in a situation fraught with conflict. Pick the people who will be most effective; set a date, time and place for the intervention; and agree on the consistent message that everyone will present. A team of four to six people is usually a good size.

4. *Decide on consequences.* As noted, there must be specific things that will happen if your loved one does *not* agree to accept the treatment plan—and members of the team must follow through on what they say they will do.

5. *Write down what you will say.* The emotion of the intervention will likely leave you tongue-tied if you have not written down specific things to discuss—in particular, specific incidents showing the problems the abuser's behavior has caused for you as well as for the abuser.

6. *Have the intervention.* Get your loved one to the chosen site without revealing the purpose. This may be extremely difficult, but it is crucial—if the abuser suspects what is going on, the whole intervention is likely to collapse, and putting together a new one will be even harder, since the abuser will be highly suspicious and alert. At the meeting, all interveners should present what they have written and—this is extremely important—should express their caring, concern and love for the abuser. Then produce the treatment plan and insist that the abuser accept it right then and there or face the consequences that each intervener will make clear. The abuser's verbal agreement is not enough. Bring a written contract and get the abuser to sign it—along with all the interveners' signatures.

7. *Follow up.* Members of the intervention group must make a commitment to help the abuser get into and through treatment and avoid relapsing into prescription drug abuse. The intervention professional and/or psychologist, medical doctor or member of the clergy can be very helpful at this stage, which is likely to involve talk therapy of some kind plus changes in the abuser's pattern of everyday life.

Plan for Success

INTERVENTIONS ARE COMPLICATED and may not be successful. Plan for yours to succeed and decide what to do if it does not. Anticipate the objections your loved one is likely to raise—and have calm, rational responses ready for each of them. No matter how much emotional turmoil you and the other interveners experience, do not let it show—confine your outward emotions to expressions of love and support. This is much easier said than done, but make it your goal in the planning stages and try hard to adhere to the approach during the intervention itself. It is a good idea to rehearse the intervention beforehand.

Be careful to stay on track with your written statements and not allow your loved one to move things in another direction—a derailed intervention is a failed intervention. Part of staying on message is avoiding confrontation or expressions of hostility by the interveners. Be honest, yes, but without accusations and name-calling. The abuser may very well get angry—the interveners should not. And yes, this too is much easier said than done.

New Beginning

THE INTERVENTION IS NOT AN END but a beginning of a new phase in the abuser's life—and in yours. Plan to take care of yourself after the intervention. This is important because, under the signed agreement, you may need to supervise your loved one's treatment. As a result, you may very well need counseling and psychological help of your own—so find it. You may need extra support from family and friends—let them know, and do not hesitate to call on them. You may need extra time for yourself, or a vacation, or time off from work under the Family and Medical Leave Act—again, make arrangements that will be good for *you*.

The intervention is not an end but a beginning.

And if your loved one refuses treatment, taking care of yourself is equally important, since you will certainly be making a big change in your own life by following

through on what you have said you will do. You will
need support in getting through that change. Decide
what sort of support works best for you—whether from
family, friends, colleagues, members of the clergy, a
formal support group, or an organization dedicated to
helping people cope with loved ones' abuse and addiction. Reach out in ways that seem best to you, just as
you reached out when arranging the failed intervention.
People supported you in trying to intervene for your
loved one's benefit—they will support you in dealing
with your own new reality.

Accepted or Rejected

IF YOUR LOVED ONE signs the agreement to get help,
be supportive throughout the treatment, whatever it
may be. This could mean you will be making visits,
sending letters and making calls to a rehab center, or
doing many drives to and from a therapy group, or arranging your schedule to be there for visits to doctors,
or any one of a number of other possibilities. You will
be rearranging your life to help the abuser—and again,
if you need your own counseling or medical help to do
that, be sure you get it. Being a caretaker is stressful and
a lot of work.

If your loved one does *not* accept the treatment
program and you have said you will walk away, *you must
follow through* no matter how traumatic that is for you.
Prescription drug abuse, like the abuse of illegal drugs or
alcohol, has many victims other than the abuser. That
is, in fact, what an intervention is designed to drive
home to the abuser: he or she is not alone in the addiction *and not alone in its consequences.*

The hardest thing of all, if you have arranged an intervention that has not succeeded, may be to walk away and get on with your life—preventing prescription drug abuse from claiming you as well as your loved one as a victim. After you move on, you will worry about the abuser, worry about what you did not do or what you think you could have done, worry about what is happening now that you are no longer on the scene—and this is unavoidable. The only thing you can do to overcome the worry—and it is perhaps the most difficult thing of all—is to focus on *yourself*, on the things that make *you* happy, on what you can find to look forward to in *your* life. Prescription drug abuse can and does destroy lives. Make sure yours is not one of them.

If an intervention has not succeeded, you must walk away and get on with your life.

Bibliography & References

"Abuse of Pseudoephedrine," http://cold.emedtv.com/
pseudoephedrine/abuse-of-pseudoephedrine.html

American Psychiatric Association, *American Psychiatric Association Diagnostic and Statistical Manual of Mental Disorders,* 4th edition. Washington, DC: American Psychiatric Association, 2000.

"America's Drug Abuse Epidemic," *Medical News Today,* Apr. 19, 2011, http://www.medicalnewstoday.com/articles/222889.php

"America's 'startling' use of mental-illness drugs: By the numbers," *The Week,* Nov. 18, 2011, http://theweek.com/article/index/221575/americas-startling-use-of-mental-illness-drugs-by-the-numbers

Association of Intervention Specialists, http://www.associationofinterventionspecialists.org/what-is-intervention/what-is-an-interventionist/

Bly, Nellie [Elizabeth Jane Cochrane Seaman], *Ten Days in a Mad-House.* New York: Ian L. Munro, 1887.

"CDC Grand Rounds: Prescription Drug Overdoses—a
U.S. Epidemic," *Morbidity and Mortality Weekly
Report,* January 13, 2012/61(01); 10-13, http://
www.cdc.gov/mmwr/preview/mmwrhtml/
mm6101a3.htm

"Chronic Pain Clinic/Interventional Pain Treatment,"
Johns Hopkins Blaustein Pain Treatment Center,
http://www.hopkinsmedicine.org/pain/blaustein_
pain_center/

"Drug Abuse and Addiction: Signs, Symptoms, and
Help for Drug Problems and Substance Abuse,"
http://www.helpguide.org/mental/drug_substance_
abuse_addiction_signs_effects_treatment.htm

"Editorial: Prescription drugs deaths demand
attention," *USA Today,* Feb. 20, 2012, http://
usatoday30.usatoday.com/news/opinion/editorials/
story/2012-02-20/Whitney-Houston-prescription-
drugs/53181038/1

Edney, Anna, "Zogenix Painkiller Fails to Win Support
of U.S. Advisers," Bloomberg.com, Dec. 7, 2012,
http://www.bloomberg.com/news/2012-12-07/
zongenix-s-painkiller-fails-to-win-support-of-u-s-
advisers.html

Eustice, Carol, "FDA Panel Recommends More
Restrictions on Vicodin and Other Hydrocodone
Drugs," About.com, Jan. 26, 2013, http://arthritis.
about.com/b/2013/01/26/fda-panel-recommends-
more-restrictions-on-vicodin-and-other-
hydrocodone-drugs.htm

Farley, John, "Regulation of Prescription Drugs Could
    Spell Trouble for Patients," *Thirteen.org/WNET
    New York*, June 15, 2012, http://www.thirteen.org/
    metrofocus/2012/06/regulation-of-prescription-
    drugs-could-spell-trouble-for-patients/

"FDA Acts to Reduce Harm from Opioid Drugs," US
    Food and Drug Administration, http://www.fda.gov/
    ForConsumers/ConsumerUpdates/ucm251830.htm

Girion, Lisa, Scott Glover and Doug Smith, "Drug
    deaths now outnumber traffic fatalities in U.S., data
    show," *Los Angeles Times,* Sept. 17, 2011, http://
    articles.latimes.com/2011/sep/17/local/la-me-drugs-
    epidemic-20110918

Graham, Caroline and Ian Gallagher, "Gunman who
    massacred 12 at movie premiere used same drugs
    that killed Batman star Heath Ledger," http://www.
    dailymail.co.uk/news/article-2176377/James-
    Holmes-Colorado-shooting-Gunman-used-drugs-
    killed-Heath-Ledger.html

Hoffman, Matthew, MD, "Prescription Drug Abuse:
    Who Gets Addicted and Why?" http://www.webmd.
    com/pain-management/features/prescription-drug-
    abuse-who-gets-addicted-and-why

Isaac, Rael Jean and Virginia C. Armat, *Madness in the
    Streets: How Psychiatry and the Law Abandoned
    the Mentally Ill*. Arlington, Virginia: Treatment
    Advocacy Center, 2000.

"Is My Loved One's Prescription Drug Problem My
    Fault?" http://www.prescriptiondrugabusehelp.com/
    is-my-loved-ones-prescription-drug-problem-my-
    fault

Kaplan, Harold I., MD and Benjamin J. Sadock, MD,
    *Synopsis of Psychiatry: Behavioral Sciences/
    Clinical Psychiatry,* 8th edition. Baltimore:
    Lippincott Williams and Wilkins, 1998.

Landro, Laura, "New Ways to Treat Pain," *Wall Street
    Journal,* May 11, 2010, http://online.wsj.com/
    article/SB10001424052748704879704575236373207
    643604.html

Maginn, Mark, "Living with Pain: The DEA's War on
    Pain Patients Reaches California," American News
    Report, Oct. 31, 2012, http://americannewsreport.
    com/living-with-pain-the-deas-war-on-pain-
    patients-reaches-california-8816508

Mayo Clinic staff, "Intervention: Help a loved one
    overcome addiction," http://www.mayoclinic.com/
    health/intervention/MH00127

Mayo Clinic staff, "Prescription drug abuse," http://
    www.mayoclinic.com/health/prescription-drug-
    abuse/DS01079/DSECTION=symptoms

Meier, Barry, "A New Painkiller Crackdown Targets
    Drug Distributors," *New York Times,* Oct. 17, 2012,
    http://www.nytimes.com/2012/10/18/business/
    to-fight-prescription-painkiller-abuse-dea-targets-
    distributors.html?_r=0

"Methamphetamine Abuse and Pseudoephedrine,"
Consumer Healthcare Products Association, http://
www.chpa-info.org/governmentaffairs/Meth_
Abuse_PSE.aspx

"Myths about Pain," Hospice Foundation of America,
http://www.hospicefoundation.org/pages/page.
asp?page_id=171115

Miller, Andy, "Painkiller crisis: Patients needlessly
living and dying in pain," DailyFinance.com, Dec.
5, 2009, http://www.dailyfinance.com/2009/12/05/
painkiller-crisis-patients-needlessly-living-and-
dying-in-pain/

The National Intervention for Drugs and Alcohol, http://
www.interventiondrugsandalcohol.org/?gclid=CP3j
hJPeuLYCFRCpnQodCAIAAg

NINDS Chronic Pain Information Page, National
Institute of Neurological Disorders and Stroke,
http://www.ninds.nih.gov/disorders/chronic_pain/
chronic_pain.htm

Nye, James, "Drug overdose deaths rise for 11th
consecutive year fueled by increase in fatal
prescription medication accidents," Daily Mail,
Feb. 19, 2013, http://www.dailymail.co.uk/news/
article-2281387/Drug-overdose-deaths-rise-11th-
consecutive-year-fueled-increase-fatal-prescription-
medication-accidents.html?ito=feeds-newsxml

Office of National Drug Control Policy, *Epidemic: Responding to America's Prescription Drug Abuse Crisis*. Washington, DC: Office of the President of the United States, 2011.

Orelli, Brian, "The Pain of Developing Pain Pills," *Motley Fool,* Oct. 15, 2012, http://www.fool.com/investing/general/2012/10/15/the-pain-of-developing-pain-drugs.aspx

Ornstein, Charles and Tracy Weber, "American Pain Foundation Shuts Down as Senators Launch Investigation of Prescription Narcotics," ProPublica.org, May 8, 2012, http://www.propublica.org/article/senate-panel-investigates-drug-company-ties-to-pain-groups

Painter, Kim, "Parent alert: How kids get into meds that poison them," *USA Today*, March 20, 2013, http://www.usatoday.com/story/news/nation/2013/03/20/children-medication-poisoning/1998237/

Palombo, Jessica, "Fla. Chronic Pain Patients Unable to Get Prescriptions Filled," *WFSU Local*, July 13, 2012, http://news.wfsu.org/post/fla-chronic-pain-patients-unable-get-prescriptions-filled

Puente, Maria, "Celebrity addicts: Who dies, who survives, and why?" *USA Today*, March 25, 2012, http://usatoday30.usatoday.com/life/people/story/2012-03-24/Celebs-and-drugs/53740090/1

Pullen, Edward, MD, "Treatment of chronic pain puts doctors in a no win situation," MedPage Today's KevinMD.com, April 4, 2011, http://www.kevinmd.com/blog/2011/04/treatment-chronic-pain-puts-doctors-win-situation.html

"Resource Guide to Chronic Pain Medications & Treatment," American Chronic Pain Association, http://www.theacpa.org/Consumer-Guide

Rubin, Lillian B., "Sand Castles & Snake Pits: Homelessness, Public Policy, & the Law of Unintended Consequences," *Dissent Magazine,* Fall 2007.

"7 Highly Addictive Prescription Drugs," Michael's House Drug & Alcohol Treatment Centers, http://www.michaelshouse.com/prescription-drug-addiction/highly-addictive/

Sullum, Jacob, "The Government's Medical Meddling Hurts Pain Patients," Reason.com, Apr. 9, 2012, http://reason.com/blog/2012/04/09/the-governments-medical-meddling-hurts-p

Szabo, Liz, "Identifying mental illness only small part in gun debate," *USA Today,* March 13, 2013, http://www.usatoday.com/story/news/health/2013/03/03/mental-illness-gun-control/1928953/

Szalavitz, Maia, "IOM Report: Chronic, Undertreated Pain Affects 116 Million Americans," *Time,* June 29, 2011, http://healthland.time.com/2011/06/29/report-chronic-undertreated-pain-affects-116-million-americans/

Torrey, E. Fuller, MD, *Out of the Shadows: Confronting America's Mental Illness Crisis.* New York: John Wiley & Sons, 1998.

"Unlawful purchase of pseudoephedrine products," *LAWriter Ohio Laws and Rules, http://codes.ohio. gov/orc/2925.55*

"Use and Abuse of Psychoactive Prescription Drugs and Over-the-Counter Medications," National Center for Biotechnology Information, US National Library of Medicine, http://www.ncbi.nlm.nih.gov/books/ NBK64413/

Williamson, David, "Durect Investors Feel the Pain," *Motley Fool*, Jan. 6, 2012, http://www.fool.com/ investing/general/2012/01/06/durect-investors-feel-the-pain.aspx

Young, Saundra, "White House launches effort to combat soaring prescription drug abuse," CNN Health, Apr. 19, 2011, http://www.cnn.com/2011/ HEALTH/04/19/drug.abuse/index.html

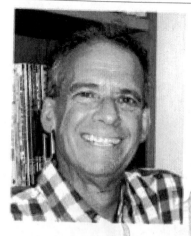

Mark J. Estren, Ph.D., received his doctorates in psychology and English from the University at Buffalo and his master's degree in journalism from Columbia University. A Pulitzer-winning journalist, he has held top-level positions at numerous print and broadcast news organizations for more than 30 years, ranging from producer of "Report on Medicine" for CBS Radio to frequent health-related reporting for the *Bottom Line* newsletter group. Among his other affiliations have been *The Washington Post, Miami Herald, Philadelphia Inquirer,* United Press International, and CBS and ABC News. He was named one of *Fortune* magazine's "People to Watch." Experienced in business as well as health and medicine, he was general manager of Financial News Network, creator and executive producer of the national edition of *The Nightly Business Report,* and editor of *High Technology Business* magazine. His offices are in Fort Myers, Florida. www.markjestren.com.

RONIN BOOKS FOR INDEPENDENT MINDS

STATINS ....Estren STAT14.95 ___

    Most prescribed drug in USA. Miraculous or misguided?

QUESTION AUTHORITY...Potter QUES 14.95 ___

    Think for yourself; deflect ridicule.

OVERCOMING JOB BURNOUT ....Potter OVEJOB 14.95 ___

    How to renew enthusiasm for working. Principles of self-management.

HIGH PERFORMANCE GOAL SETTING ....Potter HIGOAL 9.95 ___

    How to use intuition to conceive and achieve your dreams.

BRAIN BOOSTERS ....Potter/Orfali BRABOO 16.95 ___

    Foods and drugs that make you smarter..

SMART WAYS TO STAY YOUNG & HEALTHY ....Gascoign SMAWAY 12..95 ___

    Kaiser doctor tells ways to increase health and life-span.

CHANGE YOUR MIND; CHANGE YOUR WEIGHT.. Mautner CHAWEI 12.95 ___

    Scientific cognative approach to weight loss

FROM CONFLICT TO COOPERATION ....Potter FROCON 14.95 ___

    How to mediate a dispute, step-by-step technique.

WORRYWART'S COMPANION ....Potter WORWAR 12.95 ___

    21 ways to soothe yourself and worry smart.

DRUG TESTING AT WORK ....Potter & Orfali DRUTES 24.95 ___

    A guide for employers.

Books prices: SUBTOTAL $_____

CA customers add sales tax 9.00% _____

BASIC SHIPPING: (All orders) $6.00

PLUS SHIPPING: USA+$1 for each book, Canada+$2 for each book, Europe+$7 for each book, Pacific+$10 for each book

Books + Tax + Basic + Shipping: TOTAL $_____

Checks/Money Order Payable to Ronin Publishing

MC _ Visa _ Exp date __ _ __ card #: _ _ _ _ _ _ _ _ _ _ _ _ _ _ _ _ _ (sign) _ _ _ _ _ _ _ _ _ _

Name_ _

Address _ _ _ _ _ _ _ _ _ _ _ _ _ _ _ _ _ _ _ City _ _ _ _ _ _ _ _ _ _ _ State _ _ _ ZIP_____

PRICE & AVAILABILITY SUBJECT TO CHANGE WITHOUT NOTICE

• Info (510)420-3669 •

Available at amazon.com or order through your independent bookstore.

- Ronin Publishing, Inc. • Box 22900 Oakland CA 94609

Stores & Distributors — Call for Wholesale info